BUILT
TO
SURVIVE

A Comprehensive Guide to the Medical Use of Anabolic Therapies, Nutrition, Supplementation and Exercise for HIV (+) Men and Women

By Michael Mooney and Nelson Vergel

100 %
of the profits from the sale of this book will benefit non-profit HIV organizations

Foreword by
Mauro Di Pasquale, M.D.
Patricia Salvato, M.D
and Shannon Schrader, M.D.

Cover Design: Vilven Design of Houston, Texas
Cover Photo: Matt Soileau, Houston, Texas
Cover Model: Aaron Molitor

Published by: Program for Wellness Restoration (PoWeR)

Library of Congress Cataloging-in-Publication Data

Mooney, Michael, 1953

Vergel, Nelson, 1959

Built to Survive: A Comprehensive Guide to The Medical Use
of Anabolic Therapies, Nutrition, Supplementation and Exercise for HIV (+) Men and Women
Includes medical journal references and index.

ISBN 0-9662231-0-1

Medicine, Health, AIDS, Nutrition, Chemistry, Endocrinology

Library of Congress Catalog Card Number 97-076291

OUR VISION

Until there is a cure, we envision a day when wasting syndrome will have clear, practical, and comprehensive standard of care guidelines with prophylaxis and intervention therapies that are cost effective and accessible to every HIV-positive man, woman, and child in the U.S. and around the world.

To those who have helped our efforts to carry this message:

In memory of:

Michael Dullnig, M.D., for sparking this effort. His memory lives in this book.

Barry Chadsey, M.D., for having the guts to pioneer this therapy.

Preston Keith, who helped Nelson find this life-saving therapy.

To Chester Meyers, Ph.D., for his contributions to progressive nutrition for HIV.

And to all those who have died from wasting syndrome. May God rest their souls.

Special Thanks from Nelson Vergel to:

Mauro Di Pasquale, M.D., for sharing his expertise from the start and bringing Michael Mooney to my life.

Patricia Salvato, M.D., for believing in me from the beginning, even when most doctors were skeptical.

My doctor Shannon Schrader, M.D., for his compassion, support, and selfless commitment to the HIV community.

Gary Bucher, M.D., for initiating his groundbreaking anabolic study.

Fred Sattler, M.D., for listening to us.

Al Benson, for being committed to spreading the word.

My life partner, Tim Baker, whose love and support has brought stability into my life that has enabled me to do this work without worries.

My mother, Hilda, a woman who taught me the joy of helping others, and to my brothers and sisters, who have always stood next to me.

My friend Richard Wiederholt, the wise man in my life.

My friend Anthony Bianchi, whose love and support empower me.

Our PoWeR advisory board members and Body Positive Houston board members, for believing in this work.

All progressive physicians, registered dietitians, nutritionists, and exercise trainers who help people by trusting their intuition before controlled data are available.

Special Thanks from Michael Mooney to:

To my life partner Jim Brockman, for sharing his intelligence and his insight. Without him my work would be twice as difficult.

Mauro Di Pasquale, M.D., for introducing me to Nelson.

Walter Jekot, M.D, for going against the grain.

Lark Lands, Ph.D., for her willingness to lead, where others follow.

Fred Sattler, M.D., for accepting us as equals.

Al Benson, for his personal courage.

Dan Duchaine, for his good advice and support.

To Bill Phillips and T.C. Luoma, for delivering my message to 300,000 Muscle Media readers.

To my mother, who has always been there for those who are less fortunate.

And finally, thank you to my sister Kathy and my father Patrick, because if they had not let me have time away from work and given me their full support, I would not have been able to do any of this.

And for all the people who have benefited from our work and shared it with others, God bless each of you. We do this for you.

Contents

Foreword

I was both honored and pleased that Michael and Nelson asked me to do a foreword for their new book. This book has been a long time coming and is eagerly awaited by everyone who has been involved in fighting the devastating effects of the HIV virus.

I was fortunate enough to have known and helped the late Dr. Michael Dullnig, also known as "Dr. X" in Muscle Media magazine, in his efforts to spread the word about the devastating effects of weight loss in HIV and the often life-saving effects of anabolic steroids. I corresponded with Dr. Dullnig back in 1993 and after sending him my various publications I advised and collaborated with him until his death in June of 1994. He was an intelligent, knowledgeable, and dedicated man, who made a significant difference in all of our lives.

Before his death, Dr. Dullnig passed the torch to Nelson Vergel. I remember when Nelson called me asking for my help, saying that Dullnig had sent him over a quarter ton of research material just before Dullnig's death. From the first time I spoke with Nelson I had no doubt that he would succeed in his efforts to understand and apply the healing principles that would eventually make such a big difference in the lives of all HIV(+) men and women.

A short time after Dullnig died I received a call from Michael Mooney, who was independently researching the use of anabolic steroids and other growth factors in AIDS. Realizing that they had so much in common I gave Nelson's phone number to Michael in the hope that they would collaborate. On looking back my giving Nelson's phone number to Michael was one of those meant-to-be kinds of things. The results of their collaboration turned out to be more than I had hoped for.

I have watched over the years as both Michael and Nelson have changed from being innocent idealists to being veterans in researching, speaking and writing on various aspects of HIV disease and its treatment. This evolutionary process has resulted in an astounding transformation, so much so that while at first I had much to teach them, they now have surpassed my knowledge and expertise on several fronts. Today they are two of the most knowledgeable and dedicated people I know, and equally important, the most caring and unselfish. Without these special attributes their work and this book would never have been. Together Michael and Nelson have made a difference to every HIV(+) person. This book is a culmination of their knowledge, hopes, and desires to help their fellows.

Michael and Nelson tell me that I am one of their role models because of my work back to the late seventies on anabolic steroids and other growth-inducing compounds, as well as my ongoing work on nutrition and ergogenic supplements. I am proud to have played a part in their accomplishments, but I am especially proud that they say they learned a lot about the value of substantiating what they say with references to the medical literature from my work. In our interactions over a number of years I have encouraged each of them to go where others fear to tread, but stand on solid ground, and I think this book does exactly that.

Among many other things, you will learn how the judicious use of anabolic compounds, along with optimal nutrition, exercise and other treatment modalities, will increase longevity and dramatically improve the quality-of-life for those who are HIV positive. But while this book will help people with HIV learn about some important survival tools, that is not all you will get from reading it. This book, while important for its educational content and clinical information, is a testimony to what can be done against adversity and ignorance. What emanates from this book is the courage, dedication, and vision of its authors. For them this book is but one stepping stone in their journey. One that will not end until a cure is found.

Mauro Di Pasquale, M.D.
Ontario, Canada

This book, by its very name, is reflective of survival, survival of the fittest. Michael Mooney and Nelson Vergel endeavor to shift the mind-set of HIV as a terminal wasting illness, into a mind-set of health-enhancing behaviors that can contribute to long-term survival. Even though there is no cure yet in HIV disease, a life of quality and value can be sustained in this disease. Continuing education for the physician has been a fundamental precept of the profession since the case descriptions of Hippocrates were used to understand prognosis. Physicians have always been expected to follow a personal plan for progressive learning throughout their practicing careers. The principles supported by Michael Mooney and Nelson Vergel have undoubtedly added to the full picture of care for my HIV patients and have been an incredible learning experience in my practice.

This book reflects an encouraging public trend towards the assumption of personal responsibility for treating HIV disease. It urges the patient to take an active role in treating his or her condition, in combination with traditional medical treatment. The concepts in this book help strengthen the HIV patient's will to live against the constant threats of HIV's desire to kill. I have seen in my practice that using all options and enlisting the patient's innate ability to heal has helped lead to long-term survivors. Drawing on my experience and that of the many exceptional people I have encountered and the many exceptional things that they have taught me has added a new dimension to the quality-of-life of my patients with HIV disease.

In HIV disease, weight loss has been associated with an increased risk of mortality in a number of studies, and also with an increased risk of hospitalization and in the development and progression of the disease. Regardless of T-cell count, body cell mass correlates with quality-of-life. Early studies noted a disproportionate loss of body cell mass compared to fat mass and that depletion of body cell mass may start early in the illness, even before significant immune dysfunction is present. Studies have shown that as little as a 5 percent weight loss can increase morbidity and increase risk of infection. Anabolic steroids are receiving increased attention as a treatment, both for wasting syndrome and to prevent loss of crucial lean body mass. Anabolic steroids increase the retention of nitrogen in the body and promote weight gain and increased body cell mass, especially when combined with an exercise program.

Anabolic steroids are certainly no cure for AIDS, and their use, like all drugs, can produce side effects. The benefits far outweigh the risks as side effects can all be easily managed with the guidance of a physician. Testosterone and anabolic steroids can provide the following positive effects:

1. Stimulate appetite,
2. Promote muscle anabolism, reduce catabolism,
3. Increase muscle protein synthesis,
4. Stimulate growth hormone (GH) and insulin-like growth factor-1,
5. Stimulate the immune response,
6. Improve overall sense of well-being.

By finding medications which reverse the depletion of body cell mass, we may be able to add years to the lives of our HIV/AIDS patients. I believe that we can increase the quality-of-life and positively alter the CD4 T-helper and the CD8 suppressor cell counts and ratios in patients by using anabolic steroid therapy

As we slowly approach a cure for this disease, anabolic steroids may be the missing ingredient necessary to prevent the body's premature depletion of its mass and thus prevent the descending spiral into life-threatening metabolic, endocrinological, and infectious complications.

The results following the principles set forth in this book, give HIV(+) people for the first time, the power of self-esteem in this disease. Researchers are now studying the very strong relationship among attitudinal healing and immune function. I have learned over my years of practice that one cannot understand disease unless one understands the person who has the disease and also understand their feelings of helplessness that the disease can sometimes create in them. We must all confront the reality that no one lives forever. Illness and death are not signs of failure; what is failure is not choosing to live. The goal should be to live with dignity and quality-of-life making each day meaningful and life-sustaining.

As I have watched my patients battle this disease, I know how courageous they are and how much they have learned about healing. I see in survivors how they embrace life, not how they avoid death. Those who learn to take the challenge of their illness and share responsibility for their treatment have chosen a path that leads to peace of mind and healing on both a spiritual and physical basis.

No two people manage their illnesses exactly the same way, even if they have the same disease, the same doctors, and the same treatments available to them. In the end, each person must manage their life in a way that makes sense to themselves.

This book represents much of what has been learned through collective experiences about HIV wasting syndrome and how to treat it as well as about preventing the wasting that can accompany HIV disease. More specifically, it represents the fact that an independent will to live, combined with health-enhancing behaviors, can contribute to prolonged survival; even when cure is not possible, a life of quality and value can be sustained until the end. This book also teaches the patient to be informed and assertive and not be shy about telling his or her doctor about this program and the successes that have been seen. Patients deserve the best possible understanding of their problems and the best treatment combinations. Combining knowledge from this book with the guidance of the medical profession, will certainly enhance health and lead to a long and more fulfilling life. *Built to Survive* should be helpful, not only to interested patients, but also to physicians and other healthcare providers dealing in the daily battle against HIV disease.

The comprehensive scope and treatment of this subject, the obvious expertise of the authors, the interesting anecdotes related by a patient, not only present valuable information in an interesting way, but this book serves as a true foundation for patients willing to fight the fight and for physicians facing the demands of HIV disease that require immense flexibility, tolerance, and an ability to have a true physician/patient relationship.

Patricia D. Salvato, M.D.
Houston, Texas

It is with great pride that I am able to contribute to this important book. Nelson and Michael deserve the highest amount of respect for venturing forward on what is still a controversial topic.

The advent of highly active antiretroviral therapy (HAART) in the treatment of HIV has significantly improved the survival for a person with HIV. In addition to HAART, other key components must be included in treatment in order to enhance this continuity of life. These essential factors include proper nutrition and exercise, additional nutritional supplements e.g. vitamins, minerals, and protein, and frequently, the introduction of anabolic steroids.

Over the last few years, I have begun utilizing anabolic steroids in my private practice as an adjunct to HIV therapy. I can attest to incredible transformations that have occurred with the use of anabolic steroids. For example, I have witnessed reversal of the wasting syndrome, which has been virtually eliminated in my practice, improvement in libido, improvement of immune function and stabilization of the physical changes associated with the lipodystrophy syndrome reportedly being manifested as a result of anti-retroviral therapy. As people watch their bodies improve, they develop a more positive perspective. Even people who previously reported some signs and symptoms of depression speak of a better outlook on life. Improved mental health contributes to good physical health. And a positive physical transformation empowers people to fight a little harder!

The greatest controversy over the use of anabolic steroids surrounds the issue of overuse. Abuse of anabolic steroids can cause harmful side effects, including, but not limited to, liver damage, stimulation of the prostate gland, aggressive behavior, depression, high blood pressure, and over-use syndromes of the joints. However, under the supervision of a physician knowledgeable in their use, anabolics offer many benefits for the person with HIV. One such advantage is the normalization of testosterone levels in men with HIV. Low testosterone levels are a frequent untoward effect of HIV infection. Hypogonadism (decreasing testosterone function) in HIV(+) people significantly correlates with the loss of lean body mass, decreasing

T-cell count, and increasing morbidity. With maintenance doses of testosterone, hormone levels in the body can be normalized.

In addition to increased utilization of anabolic steroids in my practice, I am seeing continued incorporation of complementary medicine into Western medicine in HIV care. A holistic approach to HIV medicine is growing in importance. As a general rule, this approach is not taught in most medical school settings. However, I am learning on a daily basis from my patients that vitamin and mineral supplements are synergistic with standard Western medicine. Deleterious effects from routine HIV medications may also be treated with holistic remedies. I am witnessing marked improvement in the immune system and in the quality-of-life as a result of supplements.

Lastly, the benefits of proper nutrition and exercise must not be underestimated. These parameters are integral to maintaining a healthy immune system and fundamental for living a healthy life.

My wish for anyone using this book as a guide is that he or she realizes how important each component is with respect to HIV care. The components — diet, nutritional supplements, exercise and anabolic steroids, are like pieces of a jigsaw puzzle. Each piece, in conjunction with antiretroviral therapy, fits together to maximize the treatment of HIV.

Your courage and commitment required to follow through with the dream of publishing this book are exemplary. Hopefully, for those who read and learn and grow from this book, your example will influence these people not to give up and to fight for life.

Shannon Schrader, M.D.
Houston, Texas

INTRODUCTION

This book details a comprehensive approach to prevent and reverse the critical loss of lean body mass called wasting, while it also addresses lipodystrophy, the unusual redistribution of bodyfat that is being seen in many people who are taking HIV medications. It covers nutrition, supplementation, resistance exercise, androgenic-anabolic steroids, growth hormone, and other therapies. It is a compilation of the works of two people, each of whom bring different, but complementary abilities to the table.

NELSON VERGEL, a former chemical engineer, native of Venezuela, and long-term HIV(+) survivor, is a leading treatment advocate for HIV-related wasting, lipodystrophy syndrome, and wellness in HIV disease. In 1994, after watching friends die of wasting and facing wasting himself, he discovered a comprehensive program that allowed him to gain 45 pounds of muscle and rebuild his own health. Determined to share what he had learned with others, Nelson created a non-profit organization called Program for Wellness Restoration (PoWeR), to help others rebuild their lives and health.

Nelson's vision included the creation of non-profit wellness centers for HIV(+) people, educational tools, and research studies to validate his approach to wellness. During his three years as a community representative to the AIDS Clinical Trials Group, Nelson helped to move forward the agenda for more research into the treatment of wasting and lipodystrophy syndromes.

In June of 1998, in Houston, Texas, over 100 volunteers from the HIV community helped Nelson open his first dream facility, the 4,000 square foot Body Positive Wellness Center with a fully-equipped gym staffed with certified trainers, nutritional evaluation by a dietitian, a dietary supplement buyer's club, massage/chiropractic therapy, stress management classes, and a conference room for wellness-related seminars. The non-profit wellness center concept is devoted to helping HIV(+) people get healthy and stay alive to buy time until there is a cure. To say that his program has helped Nelson Vergel return to living with vitality seems almost an understatement when all is considered. He is his own testimonial to his work.

MICHAEL MOONEY, a nutrition industry insider, has researched holistic health since his early teens, and is a journalist. Far away in Los Angeles he had independently discovered many of the same things about health related to HIV/AIDS as Nelson. After watching dozens of friends die from AIDS, and coming from a "family of activists," Mooney found himself spending his spare time working as a volunteer treatment advocate, researching alternatives to the mainstream medical model, and educating people about their treatment options. After Dr. Mauro DiPasquale introduced them by telephone, Michael, ever the idealist, became Nelson's key support person and research partner as the Director of Research and Communications for PoWeR. Nelson's vision and Michael's knowledge joined forces.

Since their union, Michael has publicized their work by producing their newsletter and its comprehensive web site www.medibolics.com, been interviewed on *Sports Illustrated* as an authority on anabolic hormones, been quoted on ABC Television's *Good Morning America*, had articles published in numerous magazines and newsletters, including *POZ Magazine*, *Positively Aware*, *Ironman*, and *European AIDS Treatment News*, and for two years was a contributing editor to *Muscle Media*, where he became known as "the medical steroid guru."

Popular lecturers, Michael and Nelson lecture together and separately, and have collectively given more than 300 lectures around the United States. Nelson has also given several lectures in Spanish in Latin America. Their abstracts or co-authored studies have been presented at the 1996 Vancouver International AIDS Conference, the International Conference on HIV and Nutrition in Cannes in 1997, the Geneva AIDS Conference in 1998, as well as other AIDS conferences. In addition, PoWeR co-sponsored the International Conference on AIDS Wasting in November, 1997 that featured the world's leading experts on the subject.

This book is the sum of the information they have collected for HIV wellness.

Built To Survive begins with Nelson's personal story, because he is the quintessence of a person who is benefiting from this very progressive and very comprehensive approach. If you are suffering side effects, like lipodystrophy caused by HIV medications, or your overall health has been severely compromised by HIV, this book will provide you with some of the most effective, easy-to-follow information about improving your general health, immune response, and lean body mass. It also gives you solidly documented information that will help you to convince your doctor to work with the progressive elements suggested here. This book will give you the tools. Now all you have to do is not give up. Keep your own hope alive, and realize that until there is a cure, you can be healthy and strong while coexisting with this disease.

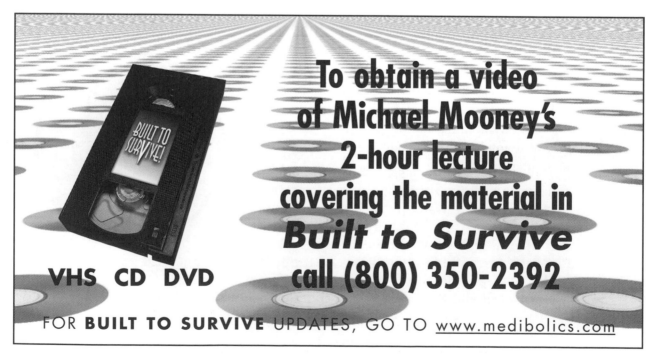

Nelson's Story

By Nelson Vergel, BsChE, MBA

I remember when I was eight years old and I asked my mother: *"What is cancer?"* She gave me the best explanation she could without alarming me, but I also remember saying: *"If I ever get cancer when I am older, I am going to live life to the fullest, travel, and do something big before I die!"* I do not know why I remember that, but maybe, it was self-prophesy. Later in life, I ended up not getting cancer, but I found out I was HIV-positive in 1987 when I was 28 years old. I was probably infected five years earlier in March 1982, when I first came to the U.S. from Venezuela. I met Calvin, the man who was to become my lover for six years on that trip. I went back to Venezuela and spent weeks with the worst flu of my life. Life went on as usual after that as I was unaware of what had started happening to my health.

Two years later Calvin called me to tell me that he could not wait any longer for me to move to the U.S. and, fearful of losing him, I sold everything, packed my bags and left my country. I had done that years before when I went to school in Montreal, Canada, but now it was a true adventure. I moved to Houston from Venezuela in 1984 to start a new life with my lover, full of dreams for the future in the land of opportunity. After getting my MBA, I found good jobs in the oil and gas industry as a chemical engineer.

One day in 1987 Calvin came to me with the bad news that he had gotten tested for HIV and his results were positive. I realized that I had to be positive too. After crying for a whole night, I decided I had to face reality. I went to get tested. When the results came back, my counselor told me: *"You are HIV-positive: go home and take care of yourself."* Back then there was nothing to treat this illness, not even AZT. I realized that all my dreams were collapsing in front of my eyes. I had come to this country three years before with the idea that I was going to make it. Instead, I was now constantly thinking an early death was going to rob me of my dreams. After grieving for days, I decided that if I *was* going to die, I would explore all possibilities first on how to stay healthy. I was extremely hungry for medical information. I subscribed to 10 of the best AIDS newsletters in the country to keep myself updated. Additionally, a month after my diagnosis I enrolled in a training program with the Centers for Disease Control to become a certified HIV counselor, when the one who really needed counseling was me. Counseling more than 20 people a night gave me the strength to continue to empower myself. I became an avid reader and researcher about anything that had to do with AIDS and health. I was still working full-time as a chemical engineer back then, keeping this terrible stressor a secret from my employer and coworkers. No one noticed, and my job performance improved, probably due to my lack of fear about future expectations. I started a search for my real life purpose, something that would fill me with passion. I knew from several research studies on psycho-immunology that those with a life purpose tend to live longer. One thing that I already knew: being a chemical engineer was not what I wanted on my obituary.

As time went by, I became more and more symptomatic. Diarrhea, anxiety attacks, thrush, skin problems, night sweats and other ailments became common struggles for me. I knew that I could not continue just doing what my doctors said, and that I needed to do something different if I wanted to stay alive. I enrolled in an AZT study, but realized that I was on a placebo (sugar pill) when my T cells kept dropping. I was also losing weight and energy. My relationship with my lover ended and I was transferred to Los Angeles from Houston in 1990.

I knew that there were more possibilities to learn about alternative therapies in Los Angeles. I was excited and scared at the same time, since I knew no one there. It took me awhile to get used to L.A. I started meeting people who were on the same search for health that I was. I got involved with very dynamic support groups where we discussed the latest treatments and alternative therapies. I started to consume mega-doses of supplements, exercise regularly and to watch my diet for allergic reactions. My health started improving; however my weight was still decreasing. (I used to weigh 165 lbs. and I was down to 140 lbs). I became more eclectic about my healthcare — I used the best that the pharmaceutical world and the holistic world had to offer. Many of my friends who were HIV-positive were against using antivirals, since they thought these heavy drugs weren't worth the side effects. I was fortunate to use them without any problems. I also realized that this virus is a very smart one. I came to the belief that maybe switching therapies every six months or so

would probably prevent a lot of the problems associated with viral resistance (mutations) and side effects due to long-term use of antivirals. I am extremely grateful about all that I learned while living in L.A. I consider that time the beginning of my transformation towards what I am today.

I got transferred back to Houston a year and a half later. I was a different person with a new perspective on my healthcare. I was more assertive so I demanded that my doctor let me take reasonable risks in my choices of therapies. In the mean while, Calvin my ex-lover and many of my friends were dying of AIDS. Most of them ended up looking like skeletons before their deaths. My ex-lover, a man who used to be handsome and well-built, lost 100 pounds (from 180 lbs down to 80 lbs) and died in bones as we watched helplessly. I refused to accept that there was nothing the doctors could do to stop their wasting, which was probably the main contributor to their deaths. I decided I was not going to be the next victim of my own and my doctors' ignorance in treating wasting. I became focused, and maybe obsessed, in finding an effective therapy to this dreadful illness.

One day in the summer of 1992 one of my friends in L.A. called me to say that they had gone to a seminar about the use of anabolic steroids for AIDS. I remember saying, *"But steroids are supposed to be bad for you!"* I remember all I had read about the abuse and misuse of anabolic steroids, about "roid rage" and about how you could get cancer and liver problems. My friends in L.A. insisted that the seminar speaker sounded like he knew what he was saying, and that this could probably be a good option to reverse my weight loss and improve my quality-of-life. I was very skeptical, but in the back of my mind a little ray of hope started to shine. Maybe this was it!

I decided that I was going to do it. I figured I had more to win than to lose. I tried finding a doctor who would prescribe the steroids, but could not find one. Friends of mine began trying to find dealers who could bring anabolics from Mexico. I also asked my mother in Venezuela to get me some testosterone cypionate and Deca Durabolin — they can be obtained over the counter there. I was finally able to obtain them and start this therapy full of excitement, fear and hope. Months later I found out that Dr. Barry Chadsey and Dr. Walter Jekot in Los Angeles were already prescribing anabolic steroids to their patients.

I was very worried about the fact that I was doing something potentially risky without any guidance. I bought every bodybuilding magazine possible. They all criticized the use of anabolics and pushed their supplements as replacements. One magazine had an advertisement for Bill Phillips' *Anabolic Reference Guide*. I ordered it and was offered a subscription to Bill Phillips' magazine, *Muscle Media 2000*. I accepted it. It took me a few days to devour Bill Phillips' book. I found it extremely helpful. However, I was still worried that there was nothing there about the potential benefits or risks of anabolic steroid use on the immune system. I remember talking to my friends about trying to find a person who would know more about that matter. Hopefully, it would be a person who was HIV-positive and maybe a researcher or doctor.

My first issue of *Muscle Media* arrived, and I read it hungrily. To my surprise and delight, there was an article in the magazine written by an HIV-positive doctor! This doctor, who called himself "Dr. X," had gotten out of his death bed and regained 40 pounds and gotten his life back by using anabolic steroids, even though he only had 4 T cells!! I called my friends in L.A. immediately and told them that we had to get hold of this Dr. X. My friend Preston spent the next two days networking on the phone. He called me back with the good news: he had found Dr. X's phone number. I didn't hesitate to call him. Dr. X returned my call and we talked for an hour. His real name was Michael Dullnig, M.D. He

was a psychiatrist on disability and was writing a book on his experiences. What a delightful, smart, passionate man. I became his number one fan. We would talk for hours every week to share our experiences. He was writing a book about his personal program. I told him I was looking for a life purpose and that I was willing to volunteer some time to help him in any way to spread this information.

In the meanwhile, I gained good lean body mass. I put on 35 pounds during the next year or so. My immune response also improved, especially my CD8 T cells, which went from 900 to 2500 cells per mm³. My symptoms basically disappeared. I never felt or looked better in my life, even when I was HIV-negative! And all this happened before we even had protease inhibitors. I agreed with Dullnig that it was unethical and immoral to keep this information from HIV(+) people and doctors just because of all the misconceptions, stigma, and hype surrounding anabolic steroid use. I wanted everyone who needed this information to have access to it. None of the so-called information-based organizations out there had anything on anabolics and HIV disease and only a very few small papers had been written about it. Most doctors I talked to did not know much or anything at all, and some were very much against the use of anabolics because of all the bad publicity associated with them. So, I decided to embark in a crusade to gather more information and to help Dr. Dullnig to disseminate it.

Things kept getting better for me. My quality-of-life got to be the best I could remember; even my mind worked better. Unfortunately, that was not the case for Michael Dullnig. While I was fortunate to have started the program while my T4 cells were still over 200 cells per mm3, Michael started the anabolic steroids when his T4-cell count had already dropped to 10 cells per mm3; normal range is 1000 to 1500 cells per mm3. Even though he was able to live a good full year after he started steroids with his new quality-of-life, he eventually developed CMV retinitis (a viral infection that attacks the retina of the eye and makes people lose their sight). He called me to say that he could not stand the thought of going blind, that he would rather die than go through the chemotherapy required to treat that infection. My first thought was to motivate him to go on, to finish his book. He called me weeks later to say that he had drawn the line and that he was going to end his life the next day on June 1, 1994. I was shocked. He was in a hurry to call everyone to say good-bye, so he did not have much time. He said that he was going to accept my offer to help him finish the book and spread this valuable information. He hung up and I spent hours crying in shock. A week later I got 650 pounds of research material via Federal Express that Dullnig had sent me. I knew my life was never going to be the same after that.

I started to get Dullnig's fan mail. I got dozens of letters from all over from people who desperately needed help. I realized how really important this work ahead of me was. I was still working for Shell Oil then, but could hardly concentrate on my work after that. It took me four months to digest all the information to be able to continue the work. I also did my own research by going to the medical library every week to read about nutrition, endocrinology, exercise physiology, and related fields. Michael made me promise that I would not wait for the book to be published to spread the information. I decided to create my own nonprofit organization in Houston called PoWeR — Program for Wellness Restoration. I sold my house. I came out at work as an HIV(+) man and told everyone about my new purpose in life. My boss was extremely supportive and told me to do whatever it takes to find myself. I went on permanent disability at work in September 1994, and was able to devote myself entirely to my new project.

I created a workshop format with over a hundred slides and invited a few experts to join me. One by one they all came to me, seemingly effortlessly. Dr. Mauro Di Pasquale, a world expert on anabolics and sports medicine, was the first to join my efforts. Dr. Luke Bucci, author of several books on micronutrients in sports and recovery was soon to follow. Dr. Lark Lands, one of the top nutritionists who specializes in HIV disease has also been a great supporter. Dr. Patricia Salvato, a very progressive and respected doctor in Houston, started using the program with her patients with great results. Then life sent me another Michael to help me in this mission. Michael Mooney, a nutritional expert in Los Angeles who was also independently researching this field, called me after Dr. Di Pasquale gave him my phone number. Michael turned out to be a passionate, knowledgeable, and truly concerned individual who is committed to researching this area and to sharing this information with others. We became partners in this mission and he joined me in my travels around the country. In our efforts to share the information that we think is so important we have collaborated on this book and several other publications. Without him, my efforts would not be half as effective. Jim Brockman, another great mind, joined us later and added even more excellent research information to our work.

After just four years of hard work, over 200 physicians, and other healthcare professionals, including registered dietitians, and certified nutritionists, are now endorsing and applying the program with thousands of HIV(+) people. At least 50 HIV/AIDS agencies nationwide have used our services as seminar speakers. I have designed two multi-factorial research protocols to test our program on males and females while using proper nutrition and resistance weight-training and we received funding for one of these studies from a foundation in late 1998.

PoWeR is now a 501(c)3 nonprofit organization. We have given our *Built to Survive* workshop in every major city in the U.S. and many other U.S. cities too. I have given a presentation to the largest medical school in

Venezuela, and will be touring South America next year, We presented our *Anabolic Hormone Guidelines* at the XI International AIDS Conference in Vancouver in July 1996, and at the XII International Conference on Nutrition and HIV in Cannes, France in April 1997, and had a poster presentation at the XII International AIDS Conference in Geneva in June 97. We have been quoted in AIDS Treatment News, POZ, Sports Illustrated, Positively Aware, and The Advocate, as well as numerous newspapers and other publications, and been interviewed on several radio and television programs. We have a mailing list of over 30,000 people, including HIV(+) individuals, researchers, doctors, case managers, and service providers. We established our newsletter called Medibolics and associated Internet web site. We helped create the Houston Buyer's Club, a non-profit organization that sells supplements at a discount for HIV(+) individuals nationally through mail-order. I have created my dream facility, a one-of-a-kind one-stop Wellness Center in Houston with another agency, Body Positive, to provide free or subsidized supervised weight-training, nutritional counseling, body composition analysis, chiropractic massage therapy, and other services to HIV(+) individuals with limited income. I have lobbied to include wellness services in the Ryan White federal funding system for Houston. We have an advisory board with very distinguished doctors and researchers who are experts in clinical applications and research in wasting and nutritional medicine. I was asked to join the Wasting Committee at the AIDS Clinical Trails Group (ACTG) in Washington, the largest HIV/AIDS research organization in the world. We also cosponsored the first International Conference on AIDS Wasting in Fort Lauderdale in November, 1997, with 27 speakers and 178 participants. And we have been able to do this with no federal funding, and very limited educational grants. We feel that sometimes all it takes in life is fearless commitment. I truly believe that conviction, passion for what I believe in, and the love of all around me have kept me alive more than all the medicines I have taken. I also believe that HIV was not a "bad" coincidence in my life but one that enriched me and made me live fuller.

We are still struggling to find funding and free publicity to be able to do this work, and have used lots of our personal money to spread this important message. We hope that as time goes by more and more people will realize how important this work is, especially now, in the era of the new protease inhibitors when people are living longer and want to take better care of themselves. Wasting is not a thing of the past. Recent data show that as many as 50 percent of people are not responding adequately to protease inhibitors and many are still losing lean body mass. A lot of people are experiencing an unusual redistribution of their bodyfat, a phenomena that is being called lipodystrophy, while losing lean body mass. Wasting still has no standard of care. Funding for our kind of work is very limited and will only increase when people, corporations, and the government realize the importance of maximizing health and productivity in a population that was thought to have no future. No matter what, I feel that I can honestly say that we will never give up. With communications from numerous HIV(+) people thanking us for helping them get their lives back, we both find this to be the most rewarding experience of our lives.

After five years of work, we are publishing this book with funds we have raised from our seminars. All proceeds from the sale of this book will help fund HIV wellness-related projects in the U.S. and other countries. This book is a great avenue for us to share with you what we've found in our search for more effective and healthy ways to enhance lean body mass, quality-of-life, and productivity in this critical illness. It took five years of work, but I think the wait was well worth it.

Peace and good health.

Jump Start Your Life with Anabolic PoWeR

by Nelson Vergel

Optimal nutrition, supplementation, exercise, rest/relaxation, and hormonal intervention have been demonstrated to be essential elements for increasing survival for many people with critical illnesses. (For healthy people, too.) Higher amounts of lean body mass, not fat mass, have been correlated to increased survival and slower disease progression in AIDS. But, how does someone go about obtaining the needed information to preserve or enhance lean body mass, immune response, and overall health?

People rarely find this information readily available through their physicians. Many physicians have not been properly educated about nutrition or the therapeutic value of exercise or hormonal therapies. Regarding the potential medical uses and safety and efficacy of testosterone and anabolic steroids, they are misinformed by an educational system that has been compromised by politics.

A study performed by the American Society for Clinical Nutrition in 1991 showed that only 20 percent of medical schools required courses in nutrition, and only one school had an independent nutrition department. Additionally, nutritional advisors that work with doctors, such as dietitians, are generally very conservative about their recommendations, and do not know about the cutting-edge information regarding dietary supplements that often times has the most positive effect on our health. Even so, most HIV medical practices do not even include a dietitian in their healthcare team.

Moreover, some medical doctors only prescribe problematic drugs approved for wasting by the FDA. Megace, for instance, was shown in one survey in 1996 to be the number one drug prescribed by over 90 percent of the HIV doctors in the U.S. Yet it has been shown to increase mostly fat content, and cause high blood sugar, kidney problems, blood clots, and a decrease in testosterone production in men, which renders them impotent. It can also promote lipodystrophy, the unusual fat buildup and redistribution that alters body shape that is associated with protease inhibitor use. Only the most progressive doctors will prescribe drugs like anabolic steroids for an off-label use or evaluate you to determine your nutritional status. So it is left to the patients to save themselves by searching for the best resources to learn about nutrition and wellness.

Learning all there is to know about how to stay healthy can sometimes be overwhelming. It can even seem to be a full-time job. But a lot of this information is common sense, things you may have heard from your grandmother. It took me years to gather information about wellness, nutrition, exercise, and mind/body control techniques. I wish someone had come to me back then with all the information I needed on a silver platter. If I can help it, I do not want other people to have to go through the long process that I went through.

Although I have been HIV-positive for about 16 years, it was not until five years ago that I started becoming very symptomatic, experiencing thrush, diarrhea, weight loss, sweats, hairy leukoplakia, and skin problems. I became desperate to regain control of my health. Doctors were able to treat my symptoms, but nothing was being done to stop the downward spiral in my health. I realized that only I could save myself from what seemed to be inevitable. I was also watching as many of my friends were wasting to death and nothing was being done about it. I guess some caretakers assume, *"Well, he's got AIDS, and that is the way AIDS patients are supposed to look and die."* Well, I want to make this statement loud and clear: *You do not have to waste away if you have AIDS!!!* And you do not have to feel frail, with low energy and no drive to live. I have found that there is a lot of new and old information now available to reverse and prevent wasting, and improve overall health and well-being.

Listen to what ACT-UP has been saying for years: Ignorance = Death. This information can be an antidote. Fortunately, after gathering all the information and applying all that I have gathered, I am glad to say that most of the time I am basically healthy, feeling and looking the best I have in years. Although this program isn't a cure, it definitely has improved my quality of my life, no matter how many or how few years lie ahead. Yes, it takes a lot of dedication and requires lifestyle changes, but with patience and perseverance anyone can do it. Now that people with AIDS are living longer, it is more important to take care of ourselves. We can remain healthy until a cure for this epidemic has been found.

Let's review the main elements of what I think you should know about wasting, nutrition, supplementation, exercise, hormonal therapies, state of mind, and general wellness for HIV disease:

1. Understand the myths & facts of nutrition in critical illness;

a. Eating more does not necessarily mean that you are going to gain lean body mass; only good quality foods will help you build a healthy body. Proper diet also helps reduce the potential for lipodystrophy. (See the chapter on lipodystrophy on page 41.) Resistance exercise combined with proper nutrition is the key for enhancement of lean body mass.

b. Taking a multivitamin that contains 100 percent of the Recommended Daily Allowance (RDA) does not mean your micronutrient needs are covered. Studies at the University of Miami School of Medicine determined that most HIV(+) people need 6 to 25 times the RDA of many vitamins, minerals, and antioxidants to reach cellular levels that are needed for overall health. Also, a study of 296 HIV(+) men conducted by researchers at he University of California at Berkeley showed that those taking vitamin supplements over a six year period of time were 31 percent less likely to develop full-blown AIDS than those who did not. Nutrition is one of the most neglected frontiers in AIDS. Many HIV(+) people do not die of AIDS, but simply of malnutrition.

c. Fat is not a four-letter word. Many of us need more healthy fats in our diets for the health of our immune systems, optimal lean body mass growth, and proper fat metabolism. Intake of specific healthy fats reduces the potential for lipodystrophy, while intake of other fats can increase it. Also, low-fat diets can make it very difficult for you to gain lean body mass.

d. Eating well does not mean you will not need nutritional supplementation. Studies show that even HIV-negative people have a hard time getting enough essential nutrients. As mentioned before, HIV disease dramatically increases your requirements, no matter how many CD4 T cells you have.

e. Because the lean body mass supplies fuel to the immune system, lean body mass is critically important to long-term survival. Total body weight is a good indicator, but knowing your body composition and lean body mass is the key to detecting early stage wasting.

f. You may be losing lean body mass even though your body weight has not changed. In early wasting, fat and water content can be increasing at such a rate that you continue to weigh the same but are actually losing critical lean body mass. Body composition analysis via bioelectrical impedance analysis (BIA) should be a standard test that you are given when you are diagnosed, just as viral load and T-cell counts are.

g. Increased fuel needs caused by fighting the infections that come with HIV can be the main cause of weight loss when food intake and other factors can not explain it.

h. Aerobic exercise can cause you to lose lean body mass, so it should only be done when you are healthy and your lean body mass is stable. It can also probably help those with lipodystrophy.

i. Nutritional education/intervention should be provided as soon as someone finds out they are HIV-positive, *not* when they are already wasting, which is generally in the middle and late stages of the disease.

2. **Understand that you are in control of your healthcare decisions;**
Physicians are trained to treat symptoms, and sometimes they may not be proactive enough to keep you healthy unless you are assertive and aggressive about your own choices. You should become his/her partner in your health-care, and not assume that they are going to take care of you without your own efforts. Physicians are very busy people who sometimes do not have the time to update themselves with the latest information. Educate yourself and bring any new information to your physician's attention. Ask a lot of questions. Registered dietitians are similar in that their methodology is generally very conservative, so they usually won't suggest the more progressive nutritional techniques. While there is good reason for the conservative approach of the mainstream medical and nutritional people, the HIV community has benefited from many things that have not gone through the typical review or approval process. And HIV(+) people often times do not have the luxury of waiting until something is proven to be effective. Finding new approaches that are effective right now can extend and improve our lives. Keep your mind open.

3. **Be an empowered and informed consumer;**
Keep good records of your blood work; demand copies of all lab tests and ask to be taught how to read them. HIV(+) people fuel a multibillion-dollar medical industry. A study in the February 1995 issue of AIDS Patient Care found that the monthly estimated cost for care for the first six months after AIDS diagnosis was $2,764 and people with advanced AIDS were likely to spend $9,098 on monthly medical costs (before protease inhibitors). Considering the expense, it is only fair that we get optimum health care. We have to demand sound proactive care through, among other avenues, nutritional intervention. It has been many years since this disease was recognized and we still are dealing with basics like lack of good nutritional advice for people living with HIV. Demand recommendations from your physician. He/she is obligated to refer you to a licensed nutritionist or dietitian covered under your insurance. Also, inform yourself by subscribing to newsletters such

as AIDS Treatment News (415-255-0588), Treatment Issues (GMHC, 132 West 24th St, New York, New York 10011), BETA (1-800-327-9893), Medibolics (310-360-0654) and Critical Path AIDS Project (215-545-2212). Subscribe to internet newsgroups like lipidlist and the PI treatment list. Also, read books like *Healing HIV* by Dr. Jon Kaiser, and *Surviving with AIDS* by Callaway/Whitney. And study the orthomolecular nutrition section of this book on page 86. Information obtained from these sources will keep you current and also give you the tools to hold intelligent discussions with your healthcare practitioner about your treatment options.

4. Engage in optimal nutrition;

To compensate for the increased basal metabolic rate encountered in HIV that tends to deplete lean body mass, work to improve your nutritional intake, especially protein intake, which is key to building lean body mass. This is detailed in this book's section on orthomolecular nutrition. Appetite stimulants, like Marinol, may be required for some people.

5. Ensure optimum supplementation to compensate for high oxidative stress in your illness;

Several studies have shown a strong correlation with taking supplements and extended life span. The rapid turnover of HIV and death of T cells on a daily basis can cause increased catabolic cytokines (protein messengers in the immune system) and free radical damage of cells. (For our recommendations for daily nutrient supplementation, see the chapter on orthomolecular nutrition.)

6. Find out what your nutritional status is;

Most people take supplements and eat a good diet but still do not know whether or not their requirements are being met. As I said before, highly oxidative stress is typical of critical illnesses like HIV disease and cancer, but we

are all bio-chemically different. The recommendations presented above are good starting points, but readjustment of dosages of micronutrients are needed after your nutritional status is determined. There are techniques currently used by many physicians to determine your micronutrient, and antioxidant status, to detect malabsorption problems, and to determine what foods or compounds create an allergic response that burdens your immune system. There are several tests that help to determine someone's cellular vitamin/antioxidant status, allergies, and gut absorption. They are SpectraCell's EMA and Spectrox tests, Pantox's Antioxidant Status Test, Seraimmune Physicians Elisa/Act allergen tests, Great Smokies Digestive Analysis tests, and body composition tests, among others. Ask your physician or dietitian about them.

7. Start a resistance weight-training exercise program;

The most efficient way to stimulate the body to increase lean body mass is through resistance weight-training. Note that aerobics won't substitute for weights. Weight-training has also been shown to improve people's quality-of-life and strength. Most of us are fatigued and do not think we can exercise. However, starting slowly and conservatively will get you started and help you adapt to this lifestyle change. (See the weight-training section in this book on page 129 for the exercise phase best suited for your energy level and disease status.)

8. Get hormonal intervention (for those metabolically challenged);

Due to the high basal metabolic rate (BMR), catabolic cytokine activity, inadequate energy and caloric intake, hormonal disturbances, and other factors, some HIV(+) people need testosterone and anabolic steroids like nandrolone decanoate (Deca Durabolin), stanozolol (Winstrol), oxandrolone (Oxandrin), or oxymetholone (Anadrol). Anabolic steroids are synthetic derivatives of the body's natural anabolic hormone testosterone. These compounds increase protein utilization for muscle growth (anabolism), increase appetite, stamina, libido, and help to produce a feeling of well-being. Although they are illegal for use for those with no justifiable medical condition, they are perfectly legal by prescription for people with wasting diseases. Many HIV specialists prescribe them on a weekly or semi-weekly maintenance schedule to prevent wasting, or in a 10 to 16-week high dose, cycling manner for those who have already lost over 10 percent of their body weight. Anabolic steroids do not help build optimal lean body mass without proper nutrition (specifically adequate protein intake and optimal calories) and weight-training. Sitting at home watching TV will not make your lean body mass grow, although rest is extremely important in any wellness program like this. (See the sections on anabolic steroids and the PoWeR *Anabolic Hormone Guidelines* on page 63 for more details.)

8. Learn, Labor, Love, Laugh, Let Go;
Dr. Barrie Greiff, formerly a psychiatrist at the Harvard Business School, believes that a positive approach to life correlates with health and happiness. He suggests certain personal habits are advantageous. His five L's of success are learn, labor, love, laugh, let go. Following these suggestions allows you to embrace life with involvement, challenge, empowerment, and fun. Approach each day as a chance to learn (be open to new experiences); labor (at something that satisfies you and brings meaning to your life); love (give, recognize, and receive); laugh (with yourself and others); and let go (release things that are out of your control). If you feel alone in your battle, you should know that you are not. Thousands of people are going through the same awareness experience. Get out and meet them. Join support groups and organizations in your area. Most HIV/AIDS service organizations are hungry for people who want to help others. Get out of your shell and invite them into your life. Isolation is dangerous to your mind and to your survival.

What Is AIDS-Related Wasting?

by Michael Mooney and Nelson Vergel

Wasting is defined as the involuntary loss of 10 percent or greater of normal body weight. It is specifically caused by the catabolism of lean body mass, which results in overall weight loss. The lean body mass includes the body cell mass, water and bone. Body cell mass is basically all the metabolically active cellular mass in the body. This includes muscles and organs (heart, lung, kidney, etc.), but not extracellular water and bone.

We do not agree with the Center for Disease Control's current definition of wasting. No data can be found on why this 10 percent definition was selected. Dr. Macallan of St. George's Hospital Medical School in London, has determined that 5 percent involuntary weight loss is enough to significantly increase risks of opportunistic infections (OIs). Also, no body composition data are included in the current definition. A revised definition that also includes losses in lean body mass (or body cell mass) and total weight loss of at least 5 percent should replace this obsolete definition, one that was created years ago in a time when there was little information about this syndrome.

When the body is fighting infection, and has urgent requirements for various biochemicals to deal with the tremendous metabolic stress it is confronted with, it requisitions many of these biochemical compounds from the body's most accessible storage area, the lean body mass. These tissues are metabolized (broken down into different components like amino acids, protein, sugar, fluid, lipids, etc.) to fuel the body's response to HIV and HIV-related diseases.

For our purpose, we will discuss the loss of lean body mass and the body's use of what it contains that fuels the immune system's defense against infection. It is important to note that there is not one single cause of wasting in HIV disease, and there are numerous possible agents that are involved in effecting the breakdown of lean body mass, including cytokines, neurotransmitters, prostaglandins, nutritional deficiencies, and hormones.

For simplicities' sake, the important consideration is that the subset of the lean body mass that is the muscle tissue is more than just tissue that functions to move the body. The muscle tissue is the primary reservoir of an amino acid called L-glutamine that is used to fuel the generation of the immune system's T cells.[1-3] T cells are cells that fight infections like HIV in the body. So the muscle tissue's role as a storage area for L-glutamine is absolutely critical to the immune system's effort to fight HIV and other infections.

When wasting begins to happen, usually after HIV-disease has progressed to some extent, there is a progressive loss of lean tissue. This can take place as a series of events over many months. For instance, a person could have an infection, like any number of HIV-related infections or even something as common as the flu. Each time the person experiences one of these events, the body takes L-glutamine and other metabolic fuels from the muscle tissue to support the immune system's response to the infection. This causes some loss of muscle mass. When the person gets well, they may regain total body weight, so that their weight as measured on the doctor's scale is the same as before they were sick. This can be deceptive, though, because typically in the earlier stages of HIV, the person doesn't regain as much lean tissue as they lost, but they do regain fat and water to equal the amount of total body weight that they had before the illness. So it seems like their total body weight is normal and everything's okay, but they've really lost lean body mass and are in the early stages of wasting. Over the next several months, this same thing may happen a number of times. Each time the person loses a little more lean body mass, while they regain some fat and water. Eventually the progression accelerates and begins to bring their total body weight, including fat mass down. At this time it becomes obvious that they are wasting, because the scale actually shows a loss of total body weight. It is unfortunate that the loss of lean body mass was not detected earlier, because it is easier to reverse wasting and stay healthy if it is detected in the early stages.

That is why we recommend that doctors calculate lean body mass using BIA instead of the traditional weight scale, which only measures total weight. (See BIA, on page 18.) This type of analysis can give a fairly good relative reading of body cell mass versus total body weight that can be used to detect loss of lean body mass when it first begins to happen, usually before any weight loss registers on the bathroom scale.

Critically important is the fact that after wasting has progressed beyond obvious weight loss, eventually there is not enough lean body mass to provide fuel for normal metabolic functions and the person dies. Dr. Donald Kotler showed that, on average, death occurs when lean body mass falls to 54 percent of normal.[4] Therefore it is of utmost importance to stop the progress of wasting and reverse it as quickly as it is detected. Additionally, it is likely that it is a good idea to gain additional lean body mass above what is considered to be average as insurance against any quick loss caused by future infections. So it may be advantageous for a person with HIV who normally is light-framed and thin to work to gain extra lean body mass.

While there are numerous drugs like protease inhibitors, and antibiotics that are employed in dealing with HIV and the different infections that can accompany it, the accessible drugs that are truly effective, relatively benign wasting therapies are limited to androgenic-anabolic steroids and GH. Each will be discussed in this book. There are several issues and misconceptions regarding wasting syndrome. The next chapter details some important ones.

Wasting Syndrome Treatment Issues

by Nelson Vergel

- Wasting is among the greatest killers of HIV(+) people in the U.S. (source: Centers for Disease Control).

- Wasting is among the top three main killers of HIV(+) people in the world (source: World Health Organization, 1997).

- Two of the drugs that are most commonly prescribed for wasting are actually appetite stimulants. These drugs are Megace and Marinol. Neither of them is a true wasting therapy. Megace is a progesterone (female hormone) based compound, that effectively increases appetite, but studies show that it causes mostly fat gain, and can cause impotence in males, excessive menstrual bleeding in females, and hyperglycemia. Marinol is a synthetic derivative of marijuana and it too is effective for increasing appetite, but without the kind of serious hormonal and metabolic side effects that Megace can produce.

- Some physicians wait until wasting is evident to start intervening. Prevention of wasting should be as important as prevention of opportunistic infections like pneumocystis carini pneumonia (PCP). Monitoring body composition periodically with the use of BIA should be part of the standard of care in HIV disease. It is vital to detect any changes in lean tissue because, as Dr. Macallan has determined, just 5 percent unintentional weight loss is enough to increase the risk of opportunistic infections significantly.

- Many physicians think wasting is a thing of the past. As you will read in the upcoming chapters, people taking protease inhibitors are regaining mainly fat mass when they gain weight. The terms protease belly, truncal obesity, and buffalo hump are used to describe what is being observed in some people. Fat mass is being stored in the midsection and behind the neck, while muscle mass and fat is being lost in the extremities. Women with HIV have problems not only with truncal obesity, but also with enlarged breasts. It seems that wasting is still present but it may be simply wearing another face.

- Human growth hormone (GH) is an anabolic drug that has been approved for wasting, but its price and recommended dose make its use a luxury most people can not afford, even if they are insured. While GH does have valuable anabolic and fat-burning effects, a comparison of the studies done so far indicates that GH does not produce as much lean body mass gain as appropriate doses of nandrolone decanoate, testosterone, or other anabolic steroids. (See

13

the comparison table on GH versus anabolic steroids in the *Anabolic Hormone Guidelines* chapter on page 54.) And while GH can increase lean body mass somewhat, it appears to have no effect on muscle growth for many HIV(+) people, as most of the lean body mass gained is simply water not muscle.

• A lot of anecdotal and research information from HIV(+) people, progressive HIV physicians, and researchers points to the fact that anabolic steroids, an economical but politically stigmatized treatment, are highly effective in preventing and reversing wasting and improving quality-of-life for HIV(+) men, women, and children. It has taken years for controlled studies to be started due to the lack of interest from the pharmaceutical companies (patents expired in the 1960s for most of these compounds). Community-based trials are the primary potential source of the data needed to make this treatment approach a standard of care for HIV-associated wasting throughout the entire country (not only in the major metropolitan areas). More than 18 studies on anabolic steroids are currently underway. Institutions like the AIDS Clinical Trials Group (ACTG), National Institutes of Health, University of California at Los Angeles, San Francisco, and Berkeley and several medical groups around the country have taken the lead in this search for validating data.

• Women and children suffer the most from misunderstandings about the use of anabolic steroids for effective wasting therapy. Some anabolic agents like the oral anabolic steroid oxandrolone (Oxandrin), which has very low androgenic potential, can be safely and effectively administered to women and children. However, it is very expensive, so many HIV(+) people must turn to compassionate use programs. The compassionate-use program for Oxandrin (made by BioTechnology General) is good. In contrast, the compassionate-use program of Serono, makers of Serostim GH, is cumbersome and requires extensive documentation from the physician, which makes it very difficult for many HIV(+) people to access. The injectable anabolic steroid nandrolone decanoate has been shown to be safe and effective in a study with women who have 5 percent or more weight loss. We are also hearing that HIV(+) women are using Anadrol at 25mg per day with success.

• PoWeR strongly advocates legislating easier access to anabolic steroids as medicines. The Anabolic Steroid Control Act of 1990, while well-intentioned, took these valuable and relatively nontoxic medicines, and categorized them as Code III, which means that their distribution is tightly monitored by the Drug Enforcement Administration (DEA). In some states this means a doctor has to write a triplicate prescription that goes into DEA records. This makes doctors apprehensive about prescribing anabolic steroids, even for serious medical conditions. The Code III status and the publicity that grew around the law created an image that anabolic steroids are off-limits for any but rare medical uses and that they are much more dangerous and toxic than they actually are when used in the correct medical context. Some physicians still think that they may lose their licenses if they prescribe anabolics to their HIV(+) patients. While it is not legal to prescribe them for cosmetic or athletic uses, anabolic steroids can be prescribed in an off-label manner for muscle wasting diseases like AIDS and multiple sclerosis, and auto-immune diseases like lupus and rheumatoid arthritis. Anabolic steroids should also be considered for their therapeutic value for many other diseases, especially diseases that involve the immune system. As is true with many other diseases, anabolic steroids that are beneficial for AIDS wasting therapy are considerably less toxic than the majority of AIDS medications.

• Some doctors have actually said that providing appropriate anabolic steroid therapies such as testosterone replacement for hypogonadal patients which may increase the patient's sex drive, is unethical due to the risk of spreading the HIV virus. HIV(+) individuals may die from wasting because of this kind of attitude. Safe sex has nothing to do with sex drive, but a lot to do with education. Sex drive is an integral part of quality-of-life and the expression of love that all people need to lead fulfilled lives. Homophobia and sex-phobia have no place in medical practice.

- Studies are showing that specific anabolic steroids, unlike anti-inflammatory corticoid steroids, which exhibit specific immunosuppressive effects, may improve important components of immune competence, like the CD8 T cells,[1] which appear to increase the potential for survival in AIDS.[2] Previous non-HIV(+) studies have shown that nandrolone, can improve natural killer cell activity.[3] Perhaps this is one reason why we have seen a significant reduction in opportunistic infections when HIV(+) people are given appropriate anabolic steroid therapy.

- Anabolic steroids also have other immune-modulating properties that might benefit autoimmune diseases like rheumatoid arthritis, lupus, and colitis. Studies with male and female HIV(+) individuals are still in the early stages, but several studies will begin to detail the effects anabolic steroids have on immune function by the end of 2000. Some of them look not only at lean body mass, but what

effects other variables like proper nutrition and supervised weight-training will have, too.

- Anabolic steroids, even though they are relatively economical and effective, have only recently begun to be included in any city, county, or state drug assistance programs available to the indigent or those with limited income. Costs for the two most commonly prescribed injectable steroids are very low. Testosterone cypionate can cost as little as $16.00 dollars per month and nandrolone decanoate $100.00 per month for appropriate doses. However, only people with insurance and a progressive doctor are accessing this treatment. Some HIV(+) people are forced to buy potentially dangerous counterfeit anabolic steroids from underground dealers (with no medical supervision) because of their doctor's lack of support when they ask for testosterone or other anabolic steroids. However, Megace is included in Drug Assistance Programs.

- Anabolic steroids are available at a low cost and over the counter in most third world countries. This treatment option is one of the few which does not have to be imported from the industrialized world, and third-world countries are suffering the greatest increase in HIV infections, and without being able to afford the newest drugs. However, in my travels abroad, I have seen that Megace is still the number one drug used for wasting and that many physicians in other countries are afraid of anabolic steroid therapy.

Megace — The Wrong Drug

by James Brockman
(reprinted with permission)

One of the most commonly used drugs for treatment of AIDS-related weight loss is megestrol acetate, which is sold as the brand name Megace by Bristol-Myers Squibb. Megace is a synthetic drug categorized as a gestagen, which is a class of drugs that mimic the actions of the naturally occurring female hormone progesterone. Originally the drug was developed to be an injectable contraceptive for women, but the drug has now found a role as a chemotherapeutic agent in the treatment of several cancers in women and men, such as cancers of the breast, uterus, and prostate. Two commonly observed side effects of Megace, increased appetite and weight gain,[1] prompted its current use for AIDS-wasting.

The effects of progesterone and other gestagens, like Megace, on appetite and energy metabolism, are well known. Gestagens induce increased food intake by direct stimulation of the appetite centers in the brain.[2] They also improve the efficiency of food energy used to produce new tissue; this effect of gestagens on increasing weight is seen even when gestagen-induced increase in food intake is prevented by restricting calories to maintenance levels.[3] So much for the good points.

What Kind Of Weight Gain?

The problem with the weight gained from Megace is that it is primarily fat and water weight, with little lean tissue increase.[3][4] Through interactions with mineral corticoid receptors in the kidneys, specific metabolites of Megace promote retention of water.[5] In addition some studies have shown that Megace *increases the number of fat cells as well as their size.*[6] This is exactly what someone who is wasting doesn't want. We should be clear that the focus of just putting weight on HIV(+) individuals is inappropriate. Studies are conclusive that *survival is correlated with lean body mass,* not total weight or fat weight. So if you want to be fat and hungry, take Megace, but do not expect to gain much muscle or live any longer.

Many Side Effects

Megace has almost too many side effects to list. For both men and women the most commonly observed side effect is loss of libido.[7] When Megace was used as a female contraceptive, it worked too well. All the women lost their fertility, but they lost their normal sex drive too! Megace interacts with the progesterone receptors in the hypothalamus to inhibit gonadotropin release in both sexes. Gonadotropins stimulate testosterone production, and testosterone is necessary for a healthy sex drive in both men and women. The end-result of lower gonadotropins in men is not only lower testosterone production, and lower libido, but also testicular atrophy. In other words, the testicles shrivel up. Finally, low plasma testosterone levels are bad for HIV(+) men and women because they are associated with a weakened immune system and the loss of muscle tissue.

Because Megace and/or its metabolites have glucocorticoid activity,[5] Megace is also potentially immunosuppressive. Glucocorticoids are well known to inhibit proliferation of white blood cells including T cells, and weaken the body's response to infection, as well as slowing the healing process. Furthermore, a glucocorticoid responsive element has been identified in the RNA of the HIV virus, so it is possible that Megace could have a direct effect on stimulating viral replication.[8] Other side effects related to the cortisol-like activity of Megace are glucose intolerance, full-blown diabetes,[9] and suppression of the hypothalamic-pituitary-adrenal (HPA) axis.[5] Resistance to cortisol is common in HIV, and withdrawal from Megace therapy could result in a dangerous state of adrenal deficiency. These conditions are associated with the later stages of HIV in cytokine-related wasting, so it makes little sense to use a drug that has the potential to make the complications of HIV infection even worse. Other problems seen with Megace include thrombosis (blood clots),[10] carpal tunnel syndrome,[11] and peripheral neuropathy.

Conclusions

When it comes to gaining muscle to rebuild a body weakened by AIDS, Megace can't begin to stack up to anabolic steroids. While some people assert that Megace has a role as an appetite stimulant, there are other substances, like Marinol, that work with far fewer side effects. If your doctor isn't yet aware of the benefits of Marinol and anabolic steroids and the problems associated with Megace, work to educate them, and be sure to ask questions if they tell you they'd like to prescribe Megace for you. After all, your choice of therapies is up to you.

Bioelectrical Impedance Analysis (BIA) and AIDS Survival

by Nelson Vergel

Total Body Weight Does Not Tell Us Enough

Most medical doctors do not know about the use of a powerful, simple, and inexpensive tool to help assess their HIV(+) patients' health. As an HIV(+) patient, I have always been amazed that doctors are only concerned about total body weight to assess whether a person is wasting or not. It is well known that although total body weight may not change for years after HIV infection, body composition changes even at asymptomatic stages. Lean body mass tends to decrease while fat and water weight tend to compensate for that decrease. Once lean body mass decreases to values close to 54 percent of normal, death occurs regardless of the cause.[1] A person could show signs of wasting even if his/her body weight is unchanged. I remember how some of my friends who are now dead used to argue that their weight had not changed at all, even though I could easily see their deterioration.

A simple technique called bioelectrical impedance analysis (BIA) can answer questions which can not be answered with the common practice of putting a patient on a scale as soon as his/her name is called in a doctor's office.

One study showed that BIA indeed may be more useful for early detection of occult wasting in persons with HIV/AIDS in comparison to the normally used weight-for-height methods.[2]

BIA — Easy to Use and Covered by Insurance

BIA takes only a few minutes to determine a patient's body composition. It is accepted as a means for measuring nutritional status and body cell mass, and has been validated for this purpose in AIDS patients.[2-4] It is also reimbursable to doctors by insurance companies. Four self-adhering electrodes are attached to the subject's hands and feet. A painless alternating current of 800 microamps at 50 kilohertz is then introduced. Electric current conductance is greater in lean tissue, as it contains most of the water conducting electrolytes and cell mass in the body. Fat tissue, because of its lower water content, is less conductive.

Once the impedance measurements of resistance and reactance are made, a third number, the phase angle alpha can be calculated. From these three numbers, plus the patient's height, weight, sex, and age, it is also possible to estimate body cell mass, fat-free mass, and other body parameters. Body cell mass is the metabolically active tissue in the body, including muscle and organ tissues, and intracellular water. Lean body mass (LBM) includes body cell mass, along with extracellular water and bone. Note that lean body mass consists of more than just muscle tissue, and that many times people make a mistake assuming that lean body mass means muscle. Realize that BIA is less accurate regarding measurement of fat mass. For instance, if one is dehydrated from drinking coffee, measurement of fat can be highly inaccurate.

Phase Angle Alpha May Predict Survival Better Than T Cells

An interesting German study of 75 patients found that phase angle alpha predicted three-year survival better than CD4 T-cell count or any of several other measurements tested.[5] Body cell mass, serum cholesterol, CD4 count, and serum albumin were also predictive to a lesser degree, while age, weight, serum protein, and serum triglycerides were not statistically significant in predicting survival.

The study analysis showed that patients with median phase angle alpha of 5.46 degrees had a somewhat greater than 50 percent survival over 1000 days. (The mean -1 standard deviation phase angle for 340 healthy control subjects was 5.6 degrees). Those at the 25th percentile (phase angle 4.87 degrees), (which means that 25 percent of the patients in the study had a lower phase angle and 75 percent had a higher phase angle, had about 15 percent survival. For those at the 75th percentile (phase angle 5.96 degrees), survival was better than 80 percent. Until there is more definitive information, it may be reasonable to accept improvement in the phase angle obtained from BIA as an indicator of improved health. (I note that phase angle alpha's importance is still not proven.)

While there are several machines that employ impedance technology to measure body composition, the BIA machines that are used most often in clinical practice are manufactured by RJL Systems (33955 Harper Ave, Clinton Township, MI 48035, 1-800-528-4513). They make a hand-held analyzer, a desktop model and a fully computerized version. A comprehensive weight, diet and exercise software program is included with each system. All of their BIA machines and corresponding software cost under $6,000. Many non-profit agencies, like the Montrose Clinic in Houston, provide free BIA to HIV(+) clients. Check your local HIV/AIDS organizations for more information. Doctors can also call a company called NutriCare, Inc., which provides a loaner BIA with their BIA reporting and interpretation services.

Appetite Stimulation: Megace, Medicinal Marijuana, and Marinol

by Nelson Vergel and Michael Mooney

Food intake is critically important for building and maintaining lean body mass. That's why appetite stimulants can be an important part of the optimal approach to increasing lean body mass in HIV. However, all appetite stimulants are not equal in their effects on your overall health and well-being. The first drug used for appetite in the early years of AIDS was Megace. The previous chapter showed us that Megace should probably be relegated to the status of the problematic dinosaur drug that it is.

Recently, noted AIDS researcher Dr. Marc Hellerstein conducted a study to see if he could mitigate the negative effects Megace has on body composition by providing testosterone to males at 200 mg every two weeks with a standard 800 mg daily dose of Megace. What he found was that even testosterone's powerful effect on metabolism could not inhibit the effects that Megace has of increasing body fat and decreasing libido.

Marijuana

Although we do not have anything against the use of marijuana for medicinal purposes, our main concern with its use is the damage that marijuana smoke can do to lungs. While marijuana's effects on appetite and nausea are noteworthy, marijuana smoke contains over 400 unusual compounds, including fungi and carcinogens. HIV(+) people who smoke marijuana have been documented as having an increased incidence of both fungal infections in the lungs and bacterial pneumonia.[1]

Furthermore, studies have shown that HIV(+) people who smoke marijuana may progress towards AIDS more rapidly, with a tendency towards increased opportunistic infections, including Kaposi's Sarcoma.[1-3] Smoking marijuana has also been shown to significantly reduce the ability of the immune components in the lungs to kill fungi, bacteria, and tumor cells, as well as decrease the lung tissue's ability to produce protective cytokines.[4]

While marijuana can also contain herbicides that are immunosuppressive, perhaps most problematic is the fact that marijuana contains about 30 percent more tar than tobacco, and marijuana smoking can decrease blood oxygen by about 50 percent more than tobacco.[5] Cancer thrives in low oxygen environments, so the tar and cancer-promoting potential of tobacco smoke should make any HIV(+) person avoid smoking marijuana. So if you do choose to use marijuana to increase appetite or reduce nausea, eat it, do not smoke it.

Marinol

Marinol (dronabinol) is the other well-known pharmaceutical appetite stimulant that is prescribed for HIV. Chemically, it is a pure version of the most well-known active ingredient in marijuana called THC (delta-9-tetrahydracannabinol). Unlike marijuana, Marinol is an oral drug that can be prescribed by the doctor in three different dosages (2 1/2, 5, and 10 mg capsules), so your doctor can titrate the dosage to maximize benefits while minimizing the rather benign side effects that can occur, including sleepiness, thinking abnormalities, and euphoria. (Not a bad side effect.)

In studies, Marinol treatment significantly improved appetite in people with HIV, while trends toward improved body weight and mood, and decreases in nausea and vomiting were also seen.[6] (Marinol has recently been approved to treat nausea in cancer.) It can, however, take from 20 to 40 minutes to get enough absorption of the drug in the blood stream to feel the benefits. That is why it is generally agreed that if you're having severe nausea that is unpredictable, you may want to use one of the standard anti-emetics (i.e. Zofran), because they can work more quickly. However, if your nausea is predictable (as when Crixivan is taken on a empty stomach), you should consider Marinol.

Marinol has not been observed to decrease sex drive, decrease testosterone, or cause any of the adverse effects produced by Megace. However, there are a few things you should know when starting this therapy so that benefits can be maximized while minimizing side effects.

If you are considering starting Marinol to improve your appetite, it is generally recommend that you begin on a Friday night so that you have the weekend to acclimate to the effects of the drug in case you do experience side effects. For most people side effects subside within three days.

Most physicians will start you at 2.5 mg twice a day, to be taken 1 hour before lunch and 1 hour before dinner. If side effects like feeling stoned do not decrease during the first three days, the dosage should be reduced to 2.5 mg once per day, usually taken 1 hour before dinner. This can also make it easier to sleep after dinner.

We have also known a few rare people for whom the 2.5 mg dose is too much, so they poke a hole in the capsule with a pin and squeeze out half of the dose. This usually gives them the right dose for improved appetite and more restful sleep.

The appetite-stimulating effect can last for over 10 hours, so you will probably have a good dinner and wake up feeling hungry for breakfast, too. We also tell PoWeR clients who want to start this therapy to try not to eat junk food when your appetite increases. Make sure to stock your kitchen cupboards with nutritious high-protein snacks so that you have healthy bodybuilding foods handy when this happens. Marinol will help you gain good-quality lean body mass optimally if it is combined with a healthy, whole-foods diet that is high in protein, regular exercise as weight-training, and hormonal therapies like testosterone, when appropriate. With the greater appetite that Marinol can give you, if you do not lift weights to stimulate muscle growth and burn calories you may very well increase your body fat instead of muscle.

Marinol Reclassified

In many states, in the summer of 1999, Marinol has been reclassified from a Code II drug, which can require triplicate prescriptions, to Code III, which requires no triplicate, and can be called in to the pharmacy.

Easy Access

Another advantage Marinol has over marijuana is that Marinol is easily accessed because it can be paid for by your own insurance, Medicaid, most state drug assistance programs, and by Roxane Laboratories' Compassionate Use Program (1-800-274-8651).

How Do Anabolic Steroids Work?

by Michael Mooney and Nelson Vergel

Androgenic/anabolic steroids are synthetic analogs of the natural androgenic male hormone called testosterone that is produced primarily in the testes in males and in the ovaries in females. There are other kinds of steroids that have very different effects in the body, such as adrenal androgens like the popular dietary supplement DHEA, and glucocorticoid steroids like cortisol. Many of the androgenic/anabolic steroids were synthesized in the 1950s in an effort to deliver a more optimal protein tissue building (anabolic) effect with less of the potential for masculinizing (androgenic) or feminizing (estrogenic) side effects that may be caused by the metabolism of the body's natural androgenic/anabolic steroid, testosterone.

The anabolic effects of the steroids that we focus on are elicited by the action of the steroids on androgen receptors in muscle tissue. The steroid binds to the receptor and is carried to the nucleus of the cell where it tells the DNA in the cell to transcribe the steroid's message onto messenger RNA (mRNA). The mRNA then delivers its message to the muscle cells and this causes a response in the cells that results in increased protein synthesis, which causes hypertrophy (growth) of the cells and the muscle tissue that the cells make up.

The different molecular configurations of the various anabolic steroids cause significantly different cellular responses, and even a subtle change of one atom can elicit a unique response for a specific steroid. That is why each steroid has distinct characteristics that make it more appropriate for specific therapeutic uses.

It should also be noted that anabolic steroids, in general, are hematopoietic (blood building) agents; they increase hemoglobin production and hematocrit.

Injectable Steroids

Testosterone

Testosterone is the primary androgenic/anabolic steroid hormone in the body of men and women. Normal levels of total blood testosterone for men are about 10 to 12 times as much as for women. The Merck Index tells us that a typical normal total testosterone scale for men from most labs is generally between about 300 ng per dL (nanograms per deciliter) and 1000 ng per dL. For women it usually is between 25 and 90 ng per dL. The normal range from most labs for the subset of blood testosterone that is considered to be the most biologically active, called free testosterone, generally ranges between 3.06 and 24 ng per dL for men. For women, the range is generally between .09 and 1.20 ng per dL. It is called free because it is not bound to blood carrier proteins, so it is free to diffuse readily into cells, where it signals the cells to adjust their activity. It is important to note that testosterone production in the body declines with age and with the progression of several diseases, including HIV.

The two equivalent forms of testosterone we recommend are the oil-based injectable products testosterone enanthate or testosterone cypionate. Testosterone enanthate is sold in the U.S. as a trade-name product Delatestryl. Testosterone cypionate is sold as a trade-name product Depo-Testosterone. These products come in various 1 mL, 5 mL, and 10 mL vials that contain 200 mg per mL (milliliter). The most economical version is the generic 10 mL multiple dose vial. Prices vary, but as of September, 1999 Depo-testosterone cost between $40 and $80 per 10 cc vial.

Frequency of Administration — Testosterone (Once per Week)

While we have seen directions for administration of both forms of testosterone tell doctors that administration should be as infrequent as every two or three weeks, studies of the pharmacokinetics of these drugs show that this is inappropriate if the most consistent blood-levels of the drugs are desired. We should note that we constantly hear people complain of a large decrease in energy, libido, clarity of thought, and mood by the time the two or more-week administration occurs.

One study stated that 140 mg of testosterone cypionate and testosterone enanthate produced similar blood levels after injection, and stated that heightened blood levels decreased to basal levels by day ten, so the amount of testosterone in the blood was basically equal to what was there before the drug was administered.[1] With higher doses the duration appears to increase a

little with another study stating that with an injection of 200 mg of testosterone cypionate blood levels declined to basal levels by days 13 to 14.[2]

Looking at the chart below, it is easy to see why a person would feel a large decline in energy, libido, stamina, mood, and overall quality-of-life with two-or-more-week dosing, so we urge the physician to consider adjusting dosing strategies. We believe that the patient will experience the greatest quality-of-life improvement when the cypionate and enanthate esters of testosterone are administered once every seven days.

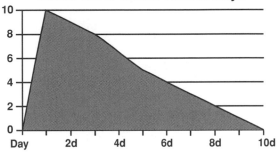

Testosterone Cypionate or Enanthate
Blood Level Versus Time in Days

Source: Schulte-Beerbuhl, 1980[1]

We also suggest that forms of testosterone not currently available in the United States like Sustanon, which is a long-acting testosterone blend, with what appears to be a more consistent release (less peak and trough effect) than cypionate/enanthate be investigated.

Testosterone is also available in the United States as an oil-based propionate, and a water-based suspension. Both of these forms are short acting and not desirable for our purposes.

Nandrolone Decanoate (Deca Durabolin)

Nandrolone decanoate is a "best" anabolic steroid for men because it has less potential for androgenic or estrogenic side effects than testosterone,[4] yet one comparison study showed that it has more anabolic potential than testosterone at lower doses. (See the comparison below.) Nandrolone, like other anabolic steroids, is not however, suitable as a substitute for testosterone for the treatment of testosterone deficiency, as it does not produce the effects on libido, quality-of-life and physical hardiness that testosterone itself does. In truth only testosterone itself is appropriate for testosterone replacement therapy.

Nandrolone's decreased androgenic potential means that there is less chance that it will promote hair loss or enlargement of the prostate than testosterone. This is partly because testosterone's 5-alpha reduced metabolite, called dihydrotestosterone, is more androgenic than nandrolone's 5-alpha reduced metabolite, called dihydronandrolone.[4] Because of its lower androgenic potential, nandrolone may also be used at low doses by women who are experiencing severe weight loss.

Nandrolone is a nor-testosterone, which means that there is no carbon at the 19 position of the molecule. This prevents the binding of the enzyme called aromatase, which converts testosterone into estrogen. While some textbooks say that this means that nandrolone should not convert to estrogen at all, nandrolone has been shown to convert to estrogen at a rate of approximately 20 percent as much as testosterone does at therapeutic doses.[3] Therefore nandrolone has significantly less potential to cause estrogen-related side effects such as gynecomastia (breast growth) than testosterone in men. Reduced potential for androgenic and estrogenic effects, along with its high anabolic potential makes nandrolone a very good steroid to combine with testosterone for higher-dose anabolic therapy.

Nandrolone probably converts to estrogen, not through the action of aromatase, but through the action of organic acids or alkalines in the body that act on nandrolone after it is converted to its 1-beta hydroxylated derivative. This means that estrogen inhibitors like Arimidex, which decrease the activity of aromatase, may not stop nandrolone from aromatizing to estrogen.

Frequency of Administration — Nandrolone (Once per Week)

Pharmacokinetic studies with nandrolone decanoate also show that it is better to administer it on a weekly basis rather than biweekly or monthly, if the most consistent blood levels of the steroid are desired. While blood levels of nandrolone decanoate begin to rise in several hours, its 6-day half-life is only about 20% longer than the half-life for testosterone enanthate or cypionate.[14] Note: The dosing information on the package insert for nandrolone decanoate recommends weekly administration. The dosing instructions in the package inserts for testosterone cypionate and enanthate are inadequate.

Oil-based injectable anabolic steroids are somewhat preferable to any oral steroid because of their lack of liver toxicity.[11 20] The main reason that orals may be preferred is because some people have a strong aversion to injections.

Generic nandrolone decanoate and the trade-name product called Deca Durabolin are sold as single dose vials in three different concentrations — 50 mg, 100 mg, or 200 mg per mL. The most economical product contains 200 mg per mL. The generic version, however, has been unavailable since September, 1998.

The Pool Effect

After several injections, long-acting injectable oil-based steroids like testosterone enanthate, testosterone cypionate, and nandrolone decanoate can accumulate in the muscle tissue around the injection site in a pool. This pooling can create a longer duration of release of the steroid, which may lengthen the net life span of the drug in the body to some extent. Even when this is taken into account, we suggest that once-a-week administration is best to maintain the most consistent blood level of the drug.

Comparing Anabolic Effect — Nandrolone Versus Testosterone

While there have been no controlled comparative studies of nandrolone decanoate and testosterone in HIV(+) people, studies so far suggest that at a dose of 100 mg per week, nandrolone produces more lean tissue growth than testosterone. For instance, in Dr. Julian Gold's study of wasting men, 100 mg of nandrolone every two weeks caused a lean tissue gain of 6.6 pounds in 16 weeks,[15] while Coodley's study on wasting men showed that 200 mg of testosterone every two weeks produced no net gain after 12 weeks.[16] Gold's study did include weight-training, though, and weight-training appears to roughly double the anabolic effect of anabolic steroids according to Dr. Bhasin's high-dose testosterone study.[17]

Perhaps more compelling is a comparative study of normal HIV-negative men that showed a significant weight gain with 100 mg of nandrolone decanoate per week but none with testosterone enanthate at 100 mg. In the same study, at 300 mg of nandrolone and 300 mg of testosterone, both steroids caused significant muscle gain, but there was a greater strength gain with testosterone.[18] (This suggests that testosterone induces specific natural neurochemical effects that influence physical strength that may be attenuated or devoid with nandrolone.)[19] There is nothing perfectly conclusive here, but these data do indicate that nandrolone probably does have more value as an anabolic agent than testosterone does at equal low replacement-like doses. This supports our proposed use of nandrolone added to replacement testosterone to increase the net anabolic effect with less potential for the androgenic or estrogenic side effects that might happen with higher than replacement dose testosterone. However, testosterone appears to have its own unique functional effects on the nervous system.

Combining Testosterone with Nandrolone to Reduce Side Effects

We also suggest that physicians consider using a mixture of nandrolone decanoate and testosterone in equal lower doses to give some more sensitive hypogonadal men the full benefit of the androgenic properties of testosterone, but reduce the potential for its dose-related side effects. Testosterone's androgenic characteristics impart more energy, physical strength, libido, and anti-depressive effect than nandrolone, but there is more potential for hair loss, acne, irritability, and prostate growth with testosterone, especially with increasing doses.

Nandrolone appears to add relatively more anabolic activity with a reduced potential for side effects. We see physicians prescribes 50 to 100 mg of testosterone with 50 to 100 mg of nandrolone per week to men to obtain better overall lean tissue retention, energy, and quality-of-life than can be obtained by using testosterone or nandrolone alone. There is also less potential for hair loss and other side effects with this combination.

We sometimes hear men tell us how testosterone alone makes them feel less than optimal until nandrolone is added. We have seen low dose combinations of testosterone and nandrolone used by a significant number of men to produce optimal quality of life, and suggest that physicians consider this non-standard use.

Oral Steroids and Risk Factors

While oil-based injectable steroids like testosterone and nandrolone are not liver toxic,[11] [20] oral steroids may be preferred by some people because they do not like injections. Liver toxicity is associated with oral steroids primarily because oral steroids are 17-alpha alkylated. If a non-alkylated steroid is taken orally it is broken down rapidly when it passes through the liver before it can create an effect in the muscle cells.

This is the reason that common injectable steroids will not produce results if they are swallowed. Alkylating the steroid, however, slows the liver's inactivation of the molecule so that it is metabolized in secondary pathways that are less efficient. This can result in an alteration in liver cell function that may express itself as elevations in SGOT, SGPT, LDH, GGT and bilirubin, blood tests that can indicate liver toxicity.

Oral steroids appear to increase the potential for cardiovascular risk because they lower HDL cholesterol and increase LDL cholesterol during use (but they are not generally known to increase total cholesterol). Lowered HDL and increased LDL are considered to be risk factors for cardiovascular disease. Whether their affect on HDL and LDL cholesterol actually increases cardiovascular risk is not clear, and there is little data in the medical literature that confirms that this effect does, of itself, cause adverse events. It is possible that any effect on HDL and LDL does not produce significant risk unless it is combined with other risk factors like high-fat, high-glycemic, hypercaloric diets, a lack of antioxidants in the diet, or genetic predisposition. However, the risk becomes more significant when we consider that a majority of the population is not disciplined in their dietary habits or nutrient intake.

On the other hand, oral steroids have the potential to decrease triglycerides by their action of increasing post-heparin triglyceride lipase activity in the liver.[7] Elevated triglycerides have been shown to be a significant risk factor for atherosclerosis regardless of LDL in one recent study that looked at 57,000 people.[21] This might suggest that oral steroids could reduce cardiovascular risk, but this generalization seems unlikely.

With oral steroids producing two seemingly contradictory effects on cardiovascular risk, much more needs to be studied before we can conclude what effect oral anabolic steroids have on the cardiovascular system, but it is advisable to take precautions, such as maintaining a mini-

mum optimal intake of vitamin E (400 IU three times per day) and vitamin C (1,000 mg three times per day) during any use of oral steroids to reduce the oxidation of LDL cholesterol that increases the potential for atherosclerosis. It also seems likely that both oral and injectable steroids' potential to increase blood pressure could be their most important negative effect on cardiovascular risk.

Stanozolol (Winstrol)

Stanozolol is available for humans in the United States as a 2 mg tablet. In both its injectable and oral forms it is 17-alpha alkylated, and therefore may present some burden to the liver, although studies on animals and humans suggest that any actual negative effect may be negligible at appropriate medical doses. Stanozolol has very low androgenic potential relatively to its anabolic potential, and while some people seem to respond to it rather well, it is still considered in practical application by many people to be only a medium strength anabolic agent. At the same time, it is considered to be a stronger anabolic agent than other relatively safe oral anabolic steroids, like oxandrolone and methenolone (trade-named Primobolan, sold in Europe and Mexico). Because stanozolol is a dihydrotestosterone-based molecule, it does not convert to estrogen, and does not increase water retention the way that steroids that convert to estrogen, like testosterone can. Its potential for other side effects is also quite low. Its approved medical indication is for angioedema.

There has been one small study published on stanozolol used with HIV(+) males that showed good body weight gains with a relatively low dose of 6 to 12 mg per day with no significant effect on the liver at this dose.[8] However, we have only heard reports of a few doctors prescribing stanozolol to HIV(+) men in the United States. We invite physicians to consider its use, as it is much less costly and seems to be more effective than oxandrolone. (See the comparison chart on page 80.)

We have also seen 12 mg of stanozolol per day appear to significantly reduce weight loss in HIV(+) men who were suffering from the catabolic effects of an infection or diarrhea. There is inference in the literature that this might be possible, as one comparison study showed that stanozolol was superior to several other steroids in inhibiting the catabolic effect of cortisone.[25 26]

Oxandrolone (Oxandrin)

Oxandrolone is a relatively safe oral steroid with a low potential for creating androgenic side effects. It is so safe that it was prescribed for many years for male and female children with stunted growth (Turner's syndrome). It was removed voluntarily from the U.S. market in 1992 when the political climate and the laws regarding steroids changed, but returned in 1995 to be sold to the HIV marketplace.

While some HIV studies show a good anabolic response to doses as low as 15 mg per day, and anecdotal reports tell us that oxandrolone is an effective anabolic agent for some people at 20 mg per day, doctors' anecdotes and one case review study tell us that some males have only a weak response at 20 mg per day.[13]

While promotional materials for Oxandrin state that it is "*13 times as anabolic as testosterone,*" this is scientifically incorrect, and a misquote from the original literature. The original text that this phrase was taken from asserted that oxandrolone is *13 times as anabolic as it is androgenic,*[22] and this number has only a very indirect relationship to testosterone's anabolic potential. Actually, these kinds of measurements, called disassociation ratios, are not considered to be scientifically credible by scientists like Dr. Charles Kochakian, the man known as the "father of anabolic steroids."[23] (This method employs the levator ani, a muscle that is not like other muscles in the body, in that it is dependent on androgens for normal function.) The truth is, while oxandrolone is the safest steroid for women and children that is available in the U.S., and can be quite effective for some males, it is the mildest of the anabolic steroids that are currently available. Because it is a dihydrotestosterone based molecule it does not convert to estrogen or cause estrogen-related side effects.

While oxandrolone is promoted as being safe for the liver, all commonly available oral steroids have the potential to burden the liver. At the 1998 Geneva AIDS Conference Dr. Carl Grunfeld noted that preliminary data on a recent large multi-site dose-ranging HIV study that looked at 20, 40 and 80 mg of oxandrolone per day showed that at the 40 and 80 mg doses oxandrolone produced elevated SGOT and SGPT, which can indicate liver toxicity. We have been surprised that a number of HIV(+) men have reported significant elevations of liver function tests with oxandrolone use. It is suspected that this happens because oxandrolone is metabolized in the same p450 3A4 liver enzyme pathway as protease inhibitors. This needs to be studied.

Although oxandrolone is promoted as having no effect on testosterone production, it does attenuate the body's natural testosterone production, the same as all other effective anabolic steroids. At only 10 mg per day oxandrolone has been shown to reduce endogenous (the body's own) testosterone production by 62 percent.[20] All anabolic steroids that are effective have an effect on the body's natural testosterone production when given at "anabolic" doses.

Oxandrolone is currently priced at $3.75 per 2.5 mg tablet in the U.S., which makes cost a consideration, (The retail price before 1992, when oxandrolone, then known as Anavar, was removed from the U.S. market, was about 20 cents per tablet.) However, BTG, oxandrolone's manufacturer in the U.S., has a very helpful patient assistance program.

Oxymetholone (Anadrol-50)

Oxymetholone is thought to be the most powerful oral anabolic steroid, and although it has a reputation among bodybuilders as being one of the most liver toxic, this is controversial. Oxymetholone is typically prescribed in HIV in doses of 50 mg (one tablet), 100 mg, and 150 mg per day, and the fact that the tablet doses are so high may account for some of its reputation for toxicity. While oxandrolone and stanozolol are reputed to have much less potential for toxicity, they have historically been studied at 5 to 20 mg doses, so credible comparisons with oxymetholone are difficult, as toxicity is a dose-related effect. It is likely that if oxandrolone and stanozolol were compared with oxymetholone at similar higher doses for the typically long periods of time that oxymetholone has been studied their potential for toxicity would be more apparent. Indeed, as was noted earlier, there was evidence of liver toxicity in the first HIV study of oxandrolone at 40 and 80 mg, but not at 20 mg.

While there is hypothesis that oxandrolone may be subject to significant metabolism of the same P450 liver enzymes that metabolize protease inhibitors, a recent study from Thacker and Flockhart of Georgetown University concludes that oxymetholone has little interaction with those liver enzyme systems.[27] This may be why we have had a number of anecdotal reports of evidence of liver toxicity in HIV(+) individuals using oxandrolone at doses as low as 20 mg per day, while we have had few reports of evidence of liver toxicity with men who were using oxymetholone at doses as high as 150 mg per day.

At oxymetholone's currently recommended daily dose of 100 mg, which is considerably higher than is necessary to promote muscle growth, oxymetholone can cause water retention, high blood pressure, hair loss, acne, increase in blood clotting time, mood changes, and most of the other side effects that are possible with high dose anabolic steroids. I also know HIV(+) men who have used oxymetholone at 100 and 150 mg per day who have experienced no significant side effects, but tremendous muscle growth, improved hematocrit, and increased energy and libido. An effective dose of oxymetholone can be much lower than the 100 mg standard prescription dose and at an individually determined lower dose many HIV(+) people report strong effects on muscle growth without problems. Recently, we have been surprised to find that some HIV(+) women are using oxymetholone at as much as 25 mg per day for good effects on lean weight gain without significant masculinizing effects.

While oxymetholone does not convert to estrogen because of its saturated a-ring, gynecomastia (feminized breasts) has been seen in males using oxymetholone, but this generally only occurs if it is combined with growth hormone, or testosterone, either of which can cause gynecomastia by themselves. Used alone, we have seen oxymetholone cause gynecomastia to shrink quickly, probably because oxymetholone can exert inhibitory, anti-estrogenic effects on hormone-responsive breast tissue.

One caveat about oxymetholone is the potential to cause a decrease in glutathione production in the liver. One in vitro (test tube) study showed that while testosterone, nandrolone, and stanozolol did not cause a significant decrease in liver cell glutathione, oxymetholone did.[11] How significant this effect may be in humans is not clear; but it does provide a rationale for those who take oxymetholone or any oral steroid to take the dietary supplements that increase glutathione production and protect the liver, including glutamine, N-acetyl cysteine, selenium, alpha lipoic acid, silymarin, and Vitamin C. (Read more about these supplements in the chapter on Orthomolecular Nutrition.)

First Placebo-Controlled Steroid Study Suggests Improved Immune Function

by Michael Mooney

When Nelson and I started our work together in June, 1994, after the late Dr. Dullnig passed away, we were a decided minority in the world of AIDS that was for the most part unreasonably prejudiced against the medical use of anabolic steroids. Back then there were only two small publications on steroid use for HIV. One was a small study conducted by Dr. Julian Gold in Australia using nandrolone decanoate, and the other a patient chart review published by Dr. Walter Jekot. Many people thought we were crazy radicals who were just "steroid pushers." Then, in 1996 came Dr. Bucher's groundbreaking placebo-controlled study that showed that anabolic steroids could not only help HIV(+) people gain weight safely, but that they might even benefit the immune system.

At the Vancouver XI International Conference on AIDS, on July 9, 1996, Dr. Gary Bucher of Chicago's Center for Special Immunology presented the first placebo controlled study of the anabolic steroid nandrolone decanoate (Deca Durabolin) with 73 HIV(+) people over 12 weeks. Results showed why steroids can be valuable for wasting therapy and supported the assertion that anabolic steroids are not immunosuppressive, but may potentiate important barometers of immune competence. There was a significant increase in lean body mass, and there was a significant increase in the number of CD8 T cells averaging 153 points. These facts are important because optimal lean body mass has a direct association with survival,[1] and while CD8s need much more investigation, some research does suggest that higher numbers of these cells may strongly correlate with survival.[2]

Although this study did not show what is considered to be a statistically significant change in CD4 count, there was no negative effect, and the trend line was moving up ever so slightly. There was no statistically significant change in viral load, but the trend line was moving down slightly. Hematocrit increased significantly.

Note that the dosage used in this study was rather low. 100 mg of nandrolone decanoate per week. For instance, a study that has just been completed at the University of Southern California at Los Angeles that was directed by Dr. Fred Sattler, who was the head of the AIDS Clinical Trials Group Wasting Committee, used 600 mg of nandrolone per week. This higher dose was studied because there is good reason to believe that it is much more effective for increasing lean body mass and that it is safe for this use. Because some of the progressive medical research community in the United States are aware of the safety and efficacy of correctly administered anabolic steroids, there are other studies in process that are using these higher doses.

Things to watch for in higher dose studies include noting whether the two slight trends of increasing CD4 T-cell counts and decreasing viral loads will increase, perhaps to the point of statistical significance. Additionally, the Sattler study employed controlled weight-training, so considerably more lean body mass was gained with a higher steroid dose and the extra stimulation of weight-training.

After the Vancouver AIDS Conference protease inhibitor combos and other expensive medicines received international press, and justifiably so, but Dr. Bucher's groundbreaking anabolic steroid study received little coverage. It was not picked up by any newsletter from the major AIDS organizations that I am aware of, and I am convinced that this is due to politics. The misinformation about anabolic steroids' safety and effectiveness has kept them in medical limbo in a community that continues to see our friends waste and die. The sad truth is that anabolic steroids, perhaps more than any other medication, can make wasting, and perhaps death from wasting, which has been a leading cause of death from AIDS in North America, a very rare occurrence. But steroids are still viewed as taboo by many doctors. Hopefully this attitude will change, as we learn the results of the numerous studies that will be completed in the future. We need to hear more about the safety and effectiveness of these inexpensive medicines.

Steroid Legality and the Physician

by Michael Mooney

The Anabolic Steroid Act of 1990 created grave misunderstandings about the legal status of steroids as medicines to the public and to physicians trying to help their patients. This law states only that androgenic-anabolic steroids can not be prescribed for cosmetic *or* athletic purposes, but the impression it created was that steroids were off limits to everyone, and that they are basically illegal for any use. This is not the case. To compound this climate of fear, it seems that when this law was passed in 1990 several of the more conservative regional governing medical organizations made an effort to make doctors uneasy, giving them the impression that they would become the object of scrutiny if they prescribed steroids at all. However, this attitude has been changing in recent years.

Testosterone and the androgenic-anabolic steroids have clear documentation that supports their medical use for numerous specific pathologies. These include various anemias, hypo-testosteronemia (inadequate testosterone production), muscle wasting diseases, angioedema, phenylketonuria (inability to metabolize the amino acid phenylalanine), weight loss, leukemia, breast cancer, and some other cancers. The scientific literature also shows that anabolic steroids may be useful for treatment of autoimmune diseases, such as rheumatoid arthritis, multiple sclerosis, and lupus.

The physician who cares for HIV(+) patients has the legal right to prescribe anabolic steroids for medical use to any critically ill patient within the same specific guidelines that apply to numerous other medications used by critically ill patients.

For instance, if a patient measures at the low end of normal total testosterone (or below) or suffers from the symptoms of hypogonadism (low testosterone production), such as impotence, testosterone replacement is indicated. One study showed that the standard testosterone replacement dose of 100 mg per week (or 200 mg every two weeks) for HIV-negative men was inadequate for weight-gain in HIV(+) progressed men.[1] In HIV disease there is hormonal insensitivity, as was suggested by data provided in a study by Judith Rabkin, Ph.D., of New York, where she showed that HIV(+) hypogonadal men generally needed a higher testosterone replacement dose than the standard dose for HIV-negative hypogonadal men to experience the normal quality-of-life benefits. As described in the *Anabolic Hormone Guidelines* section, Dr. Rabkin found that her subjects needed to be given 400 mg every two weeks to respond favorably.[2]

In 1988, frequently published endocrinologist Dr. Adrian Dobs of Johns Hopkins noted that about 50 percent of HIV(+) men are hypo-gonadal.[3] Dr. Steven Grinspoon found a similar situation with women.[5] When we consider this and Dr. Rabkin's data, perhaps as much as half of HIV(+) men and women need replacement testosterone, and men may need doses of testosterone that will bring them into the high range of blood testosterone measurement or slightly above. The physician should measure testosterone, but also consider whether the patient is exhibiting the classic symptoms of hypo-testosteronemia (fatigue, lack of libido, sexual dysfunction, depression, muscle loss, and lack of appetite) to determine whether it is appropriate to administer testosterone replacement therapy. Monitoring both the patient's subjective feelings about their symptoms and their testosterone blood levels two or three days after the fourth weekly injection will confirm whether the therapy is appropriate.

We also know knowledgeable doctors who do not measure testosterone because the measurements do not always mirror the patient's condition. Impotence, for instance, is a valid reason to prescribe testosterone, and we know doctors who prescribe testosterone for this indication when no weight loss is present. Often the person's response shows them that testosterone therapy is correct, regardless of the measurements.

Progressive Uses

The anabolic steroid analogs of testosterone, like nandrolone, oxandrolone, stanozolol, and oxymetholone are not appropriate for androgen replacement therapy by themselves, as they do not provide all of the characteristics that are necessary for normal androgen function. Their best use is as adjuncts to the use of testosterone as the fundamental androgen. They are generally used for improving lean body mass for people who have measurable loss of lean body mass; however, the most progressive physicians in several of the major metropolitan areas have been using anabolic steroids proactively to thin patients before

wasting occurs to improve lean body mass so that there is a sufficient reserve of lean body mass in case the patient suffers an opportunistic infection and experiences a rapid loss of lean body mass. This steroid-induced extra lean body mass can act as a buffer so that the patient doesn't ever fall into the danger zone as outlined by Dr. Donald Kotler, where he showed that loss of lean body mass to 54 percent of normal equals death.[4]

An example of this would be a male who has always weighed 140 pounds at a height of 6 feet. This person is below the bottom of normal on the Metropolitan Life Insurance table. This person would have much better chances of surviving a catabolic (muscle-destroying) infection, that might cause a significant amount of weight loss, if he weighed 170 pounds. The primary consideration here is the person's overall health and ability to withstand infection-induced weight loss.

Cautious physicians are unlikely to employ the more controversial and aggressive uses of anabolic steroids if they feel that they might be challenged legally. These physicians may choose to restrict their use of anabolic steroids to oxandrolone combined with testosterone replacement, as oxandrolone is the only steroid that is specifically indicated for "failure to gain or maintain normal weight." However, in the major metropolitan areas, where numerous physicians are known to prescribe testosterone and anabolic steroids to hundreds or thousands of HIV(+) people, there is little likelihood of any legal problem, even though for steroids other than oxandrolone, weight gain is an off-label use. We know of doctors in each of the major cities who employ anabolic steroids very progressively, sometimes using very high doses and unusual combinations of different steroids that they have learned to tailor for specific patient needs. We are not aware of any physician in the United States who has ever been reprimanded for prescribing anabolic steroids for legitimate use in HIV therapy.

The use of anabolic steroids is currently being investigated in over a dozen studies funded by government and medical agencies, so we are fast approaching the day when we will see the kind of broad range acceptance that will yield an understanding that testosterone and anabolic steroids are a major part of the standard of care for HIV and HIV-related wasting. We believe that any physician in this country can prescribe anabolic steroids within the context of the guidelines we feature in this book without repercussion from any government agency or medical board. After all, HIV is a critical illness.

An Initiative: New Directions for Wasting Research from Program for Wellness Restoration (PoWeR)

By Nelson Vergel and Michael Mooney

Program for Wellness Restoration (PoWeR) is the only community-based, national AIDS research organization that focuses on empowering HIV(+) people and their physicians with information about a comprehensive program to increase lean body mass for improved survival and immune function. Our unique program incorporates the use of enhanced nutrition, micronutrient supplementation, resistance weight-training, and androgenic-anabolic steroids and other hormonal therapies.

We, at PoWeR, the community of people with HIV and AIDS we serve, and the physicians and researchers we work with, have recognized for several years that the issues of quality-of-life and overall health addressed by our approach are crucial to people living with HIV and AIDS.

Program for Wellness Restoration has utilized over 12 years of real-world experience in designing anabolic steroid guidelines used to treat AIDS associated wasting in clinical settings. Our guidelines are in use by more than one hundred physicians and medical groups throughout this country and in Canada, most notably by Gordon Sanford, P.A., formerly of the Conant Medical Group in San Francisco; The ONCOL Medical Group headed by Dr.

Adan Rios in Houston; Dr. Corklin Steinhart at Mercy Hospital in Miami; Dr. Douglas Dieterich of New York City; and Dr. Patricia Salvato of Houston.

Several wasting reversal or prevention studies are currently underway that use nandrolone decanoate, Megace and testosterone combinations, oxymetholone, oxandrolone, or Serostim GH. We think that it is time for the research community involved in these studies to engage in an open dialogue to share experiences and maximize the use of resources without overlapping in their research efforts. We raise the challenge to the AIDS Clinical Trials Group, AMFAR, CRIA and other organizations in the AIDS research community to seize the initiative in this area and in a coordinated manner run community-based clinical trials to explore the intriguing possibilities raised by our 12 years of peer-driven experience.

Wasting is not a thing of the past, and research in this area should continue because even those people who benefit from the use of the new protease inhibitor combinations have a difficult time gaining back healthy lean body mass. Recently, Dr. Deeks of the University of California at San Francisco has shown that as much as 50 percent of the HIV population does not fully benefit from protease inhibitor therapy. As you will read, protease inhibitor combinations may increase weight, but the weight is primarily fat. There are also some data that suggest that at least 26 percent of the people are still losing lean body mass while on protease combination therapies.[1] What has been done so far in the area of research about the clinical application of anabolic steroids for HIV disease? A few small studies show some promising results.

Anabolic Hormones and AIDS:

As many of us know, we need a lot more controlled studies of anabolic steroid applications in AIDS than we have right now. However, as of early 1999 there have been several placebo-controlled anabolic steroid studies, that compared one group of subjects who were using an anabolic steroid to another group of subjects who weren't. The trend continues as we are seeing other studies and publications of anecdotal experiences by more and more researchers and physicians around the world. A brief review of only a little of the data follows.

Testosterone Undecanoate

Jeantils published a small study in which oral testosterone undecanoate (available in Europe, but not in the U.S.) was given for two months to four HIV(+) patients at a dosage of 40 mg three times daily.[2] No side effects were noted. Assessment of liver enzymes showed no disturbance. Weight increased by an average of 14.8 percent (11.2 lbs). The average body mass index was increased by 13.5 percent. Blood albumin levels (a good marker for reduced wasting) increased by 18.4 percent. Beta-2 microglobulin (a marker for immune activation) decreased by 34 percent. Total lymphocytes increased by 9 percent (no subset given).

Winstrol (stanozolol)

A small study that used stanozolol, an oral anabolic steroid available in the U.S., was performed by Joseph Berger, M.D.[3] The study involved three HIV(+) males taking AZT with

CD4 counts of 165 cells per cu mm, 39 cells per cubic millimeter, and 206 cells per cubic millimeter, respectively. Their creatine kinase (CK) values were abnormally low, which indicated signs of myopathy (muscle weakness). They had all lost over 10 percent of their normal body weight. They also showed signs of fatigue. Two were given stanozolol, 2 mg orally three times per day for one month, and one required 4 mg three times per day to effect a gain in weight. (Note: Illicit use doses for athletes can be much higher.) All three patients showed increased weight (e.g. 10.25 pounds average in 10 weeks) and energy levels, with no significant side effects. No immunological markers were assessed, but quality-of-life (QOL) measures increased significantly.

Testosterone Enanthate

A study performed in 1993 by Judith Rabkin, Ph.D., and Richard Rabkin, M.D., at the New York State Psychiatric Institute was designed to determine whether testosterone therapy influences sexual dysfunction, mood, energy, and appetite among hypogonadal HIV(+) men with significant immune suppression (CD4 < 400 cells per mm).[4] Forty-one men entered the study and 37 completed at least eight weeks of treatment. Hormones like LH, FSH, prolactin, and total serum testosterone were assessed at baseline along with immune parameters (T cell panel, CBC, and others). Appetite, libido, mood, and energy improved significantly after the treatments (which consisted of biweekly injections of testosterone cypionate at a starting dose of 100 mg, increasing by 100 mg up to 400 mg at the end of the study). Only six subjects reported any side effects; among those were irritability (2), feeling hyper (2), feeling overly assertive (2), and hair loss (2). CD4 cell counts did not change significantly during the 15 weeks of the study. No lean body mass measurements were taken. Dr. Judith Rabkin stated in personal correspondence that the HIV(+) hypogonadal men in her study appeared to need testosterone enanthate at a dose of 400 mg every two weeks to get normal quality-of-life barometers. We revisit Dr. Rabkin's work in the *Anabolic Hormone Guidelines* chapters of this book, and discuss what appears to cause the need for higher testosterone replacement doses than what is standard for HIV-negative men.

Testosterone Combined with Nandrolone

Barry Chadsey, M.D., an HIV(+) Los Angeles physician, a former football player and bodybuilder, used anabolic steroids to treat the effects of wasting with over 100 of his patients over nine years. Many of his patients gained 20 to 30 pounds.[6] He also saw significant improvements in certain T-cell counts in his patients. About three-quarters of his patients experienced increases in their CD8 counts and 40 percent experienced increases in CD4 counts. Dr. Chadsey was noted for using a cycling strategy with testosterone cypionate and nandrolone decanoate in a pyramid style escalating/de-escalating mode over 12 weeks, which is the format the PoWeR cycle is modeled after. (See the PoWeR cycle in the *Anabolic Hormone Guidelines* chapter on page 63.)

Similar benefits have also been reported in a paper published by Walter Jekot, M.D., a Los Angeles doctor who pioneered anabolic steroid therapy for AIDS.[7] Dr. Jekot emphasized that those patients who accompanied anabolic steroid treatment with the use of vitamin supplements, a nutrient-rich diet, and moderate resistance exercise seem to be the best responders.

Testosterone Enanthate

Notably, the first controlled study on high dose testosterone enanthate supplementation with normal HIV-negative men was published in the New England Journal of Medicine on July 4, 1996.[8] This study employed 600 mg of testosterone enanthate per week for 10 weeks, and was controlled for weight-training. Those who were given testosterone but did not lift weights at all gained more lean mass (7 lb) than those who trained with weights but were not given testosterone (4.4 lb). The testosterone group who didn't exercise also gained almost as much strength as the group who only exercised. Those who lifted weights and were given testosterone gained almost twice as much lean mass as the testosterone with no exercise group, which amounted to over 13 pounds, and experienced significantly greater increases in strength in the squat and bench press than the other groups. The authors did not detect any effect on behavior (no roid rage) or liver problems.

Comment: It is important to note that until the publication of this study the position of the conservative medical community was that testosterone alone or anabolic steroids in general haven't been proven to increase lean body mass or strength and shouldn't necessarily be used for HIV-associated wasting. This study makes obvious the fact that anabolic steroids do increase lean body mass, that supraphysiologic (very high) doses work better than lower doses like the 100 mg per week that was used in many previous studies, and that including weight-training produces significantly more increase in lean body mass.

Testosterone Combined with Nandrolone and Oxandrolone

A study presented by Dr. Patricia Salvato of Houston's ONCOL Medical Group at the Second International Conference on Nutrition and HIV in Cannes, France, in April 1997, showed that 20 subjects who were using the PoWeR program, which consists of 12 weeks of high doses of nandrolone decanoate and testosterone cypionate (700 mg per week total of the two compounds during the middle of the 12 weeks), effectively reversed wasting with an average weight gain of 13 pounds (8.02 percent).[17] Serum albumin, a marker which decreases in wasting, increased by 23 percent. No liver toxicity or adverse effects were observed. Quality-of-life as assessed by a questionnaire was improved by 188.75 percent. Although other studies have shown benefit from the use of oxandrolone at 20 mg per day, this study showed that 20 mg per day of oxandrolone had little effect (<1 percent weight increase) on reversing wasting in patients who had lost over 10 percent of their normal body weight. Also, this study showed that adding 20 mg per day of oxandrolone to the PoWeR cycle did not add any additional benefit.

Oxandrolone

While studies on oxandrolone alone at 20 mg per day have generally shown good gains in LBM, the tightly controlled Strawford study showed that this dose of oxandrolone combined with testosterone at 100 mg per week and weight training is perhaps an optimal way to employ oxandrolone. Subjects using this combination gained an average of 15.18 pounds of LBM.[18]

Nandrolone Decanoate

Dr. Julian Gold, et al. of Australia, reported in his 16-week study that even with very low dose nandrolone (100 mg every two weeks), lean body mass and quality-of-life improved significantly (6.6 lbs.) in wasting HIV patients with no negative effect on CD4 lymphocytes.[9] Dr. Gold was a trailblazer, as his study included nutritional assessment and suggestions for weight training before anyone else had done this. We applaud Dr. Gold.

As mentioned earlier, at the XI International AIDS Conference (Vancouver) Dr. Gary Bucher, of Chicago's Center for Special Immunology, presented his placebo-controlled study of the anabolic steroid nandrolone (Deca Durabolin) at 100 mg per week for 12 weeks with 73 HIV patients.[10] This study showed excellent results which supported the need for more studies with nandrolone decanoate.

At the Bethesda NIH Conference on May 20, 1997, Dr. Marc Hellerstein said that about 50 percent of his HIV patients in San Francisco do not produce adequate testosterone. His team concluded a study that employed nandrolone decanoate that showed an 11.88 pound increase in lean body mass in 12 weeks. Nandrolone decreased lipogenesis (fat generation) significantly (nutrients tended to contribute to lean tissue more than to fat tissue). Improvements in strength, endurance, and quality-of-life paralleled body composition changes.[11]

Dr. Fred Sattler of the University of Southern California at Los Angeles recently published the results of his high dose (600 mg per week) nandrolone decanoate study that compared nandrolone alone to nandrolone with weight training with 30 HIV(+) males.[18] Both groups gained strength and muscle size, with the group that trained with weights gaining significantly more strength and LBM. This study showed that even without weight training high dose nandrolone can increase LBM and muscle size and strength.

Testosterone Combined with Megace

Also at the Bethesda NIH Conference, Dr. Hellerstein presented the results of a study that investigated combining Megace (800 mg per day) with testosterone (either a 200 mg injection every other week or a Testoderm testosterone patch or placebo). He concluded that the great majority of weight gain in all the Megace-treated groups, with or without testosterone, was composed of fat.

Serostim Human Growth Hormone (GH) And IGF-1

Also at the Bethesda NIH Conference, Dr. Morris Schambelan of San Francisco General Hospital summarized the results of studies on Serostim GH, with and without IGF-1. The goal of one study was to assess whether a combination approach could reduce the cost of GH therapy. Administration of GH by itself at 6 mg per day resulted in an average weight gain of 3.2 lbs after 12 weeks. (Note: 1 mg of GH equals about 3 IU.) This consisted of a 6.6 lb lean body mass increase and 3.4 lb fat loss. A quarter dose (1.4 mg per day) gave a third as much lean body mass increase as the 6 mg dose. A dose of 1.4 mg per day of GH plus IGF-1 at 10 mg per day resulted in a 6.6 lb lean body mass gain. A dose of 0.7 mg per day of GH plus IGF-1 at 10 mg per day resulted in a third of that at 2.2 lb of lean body mass. Another study by Lee of Baylor College in Houston, using .68 mg of GH per day with 10 mg per day of IGF-1, showed no net anabolic effect after 12 weeks. Apparently a threshold amount of GH is required for an effect on LBM.

However, whether the LBM gained from the use of GH includes much muscle tissue is controversial. For more details see the section on growth hormone in the *Anabolic Hormone Guidelines* section.

Anadrol (oxymetholone)

A study published in the British Journal of Nutrition showed that oxymetholone, perhaps the most powerful oral anabolic steroid, improved lean muscle mass with what appeared to be no significant side effects in HIV(+) men and women.[12] Oxymetholone, which is sold in the U.S. as Anadrol-50, was given for 30 weeks at a 150 mg daily dose. Weight gain averaged 14.5 percent of body weight (18 lbs.), which is significant because no controlled exercise program was instituted, and it is known that anabolic steroids exert their greatest effect when weight-lifting is employed. Notably, even when patients were burdened with AIDS-related infections, they continued to gain weight on oxymetholone. Caution: 150 mg is a very high dose of this very powerful steroid.

While oxymetholone is considered to be a powerful steroid with a high potential for side effects, the subjects were reported to have no significant problems with liver function, water retention, virilization, and several side effects thought to be associated with its use. The study didn't look at CD8 T-cell counts, which appear to be more correlative with survival than CD4 T cells, which were not correlative with weight gain in this study.

We note here that the 150 mg daily dose is three times what many bodybuilders or powerlifters would use and 30 weeks is considerably longer than they would generally use this drug. However, our observation is that bodybuilders and powerlifters often combine oxymetholone with other strong steroids, and it may be that this promotes the potential for side effects. Used alone the potential for problems may be somewhat reduced, especially at lower doses.

Anabolic Steroid/AIDS Studies Needed

While there have been other studies than the few that we have described above, it is clear that a lot more needs to be done in the area of assessing the effect of anabolic steroids on the health and well-being of HIV(+) people. Anabolic steroid use is rapidly becoming part of standard of care as an off-label use. Anabolic steroids, like testosterone and nandrolone decanoate, are among the most economical of all treatments used in AIDS for their specific purpose.

Reasons for lack of research in this area are numerous: lack of understanding, stigma, and fear of side effects. In addition, studies for unpatentable medicines have a difficult time finding funds. Other problems include the belief that GH, an overly-expensive therapy, which studies show to be less effective than anabolic steroids for lean body mass gains, should be used as the sole compound for wasting reversal; fear that steroids may be immunosuppressive; fear that they induce Kaposi's Sarcoma; fear of abuse; perception from doctors that anabolic steroids are only used for cosmetic purposes; and a belief that they can not be used by women and children.

Questions to Be Answered

We at PoWeR have written two comprehensive clinical studies with the help of physicians. These studies will evaluate the use of anabolic steroids for lean body mass gains and modulation of immune response. They include nutritional assessment/intervention, anabolic steroids, supervised resistance weight-training, immune measurements, and body composition measurements for 30 HIV(+) patients. However, there are many questions that need to be answered in other studies yet to be designed.

Among the many questions that we think should be answered by research studies in this area are:

1. What effect do (higher dose) anabolic steroids have on viral load, if any?

2. What is the most appropriate strategy for application of anabolic steroids to maximize body cell mass gains and minimize any potential long-term effects: maintenance (constant dose, weekly, or biweekly application) or cycling, (escalating/de-escalating dosing plus stacking of two or more compounds which may act synergistically in cycles with a rest period in-between cycles), or a combination of maintenance testosterone with cycled anabolic steroids for periodic increases in growth?

3. What is the best time to intervene to prevent any loss of lean body mass? A study performed in Germany showed that phase angle alpha, one of the variables calculated from BIA, may be one of the best single predictors of survival (better than CD4 T cells) of 12 studied parameters.[13] Phase angle alpha increases with increasing body cell mass. A study designed to show any correlation between anabolic steroid therapy and increases in phase angle alpha might help to answer questions about the chance that anabolic steroids might increase survival in AIDS.

4. What is the effect of body weight above normal Metropolitan Life Insurance recommendations on long-term survival? A cohort study that includes current clinical data from clinical practices around the country could be designed for this purpose.

5. What is the effect of anabolic steroids on CD4s and CD8 subsets at various doses? Dr. Gary Bucher's presentation at the Vancouver AIDS Conference (Abstract Mo.B.423) showed a significant increase in CD8s while using low-dose nandrolone. Our experience with over 3,000 people also shows this effect for a majority of people.

6. What is the effect of anabolic steroids on cytokines like IL-1, IL-6, and tumor necrosis factor? One in vitro study showed a reduction in IL-1 with testosterone.[14]

7. What is the effect of anabolic steroids on T-cell apoptosis (programmed death of T cells)? An abstract from Germany showed that testosterone decreased apoptosis by 52 percent in an HIV(+) male.[15] This should be looked at to determine if it is beneficial. Is this part of the reason why patients with hypogonadism tend to show decreased survival?[16]

8. What are the best guidelines for females? Drugs like stanozolol, oxandrolone, or methenolone (Primobolan) (not available in the United States) could play a major role in maximizing anabolic effects while minimizing virilization for use by females.

9. What is the best program for pediatrics? Again, oxandrolone or GH used alone or combinations of oxandrolone and GH may be an answer to preventing/reversing wasting in this population without stunting their growth.

10. What would happen if we combine cytokine inhibitors like thalidomide with anabolic steroids, especially in patients with active MAC, CMV, diarrhea of unknown origin, or other opportunistic infections?

11. What are the long-term effects of anabolic steroid use on the hypothalamic-pituitary-gonadal axis (HPGA) of HIV(+) people?

12. Is cycling an appropriate way to administer steroids or should patients be on low doses of anabolic steroids and testosterone continuously?

13. What is the effect of using a high-protein diet and supplements like L-glutamine (shown to be immune-enhancing) with anabolic steroid use?

14. What is the effect of using a diet rich in specific fatty acids with anabolic steroid therapy?

15. What are the best anabolic steroids to use in HIV disease: nandrolone decanoate, stanozolol (Winstrol), all testosterones, oxandrolone (Oxandrin), or oxymetho-lone (Anadrol) and what are cost-effective combinations with good risk/benefit ratios?

16. How effective are the use of Clomid, human chorionic gonadotropin (HCG), and/or anti-aromatases like Arimidex to restore testicular size and testosterone production after anabolic steroid/testosterone therapy? What is the best dosing regime?

17. What are the best guidelines for bedridden patients who are wasting? This population is the one with the most imperative need for treatment and yet is not included in research in this field.

18. What effects do testosterone, other anabolic steroids, and GH have on lipodystrophy, the unusual redistribution of bodyfat seen in people who are using protease inhibitors?

19. Do anabolic steroids prevent, reduce, or reverse the truncal obesity seen in lipodystrophy syndrome?

We believe that studies involving anabolic steroids will deliver more optimal results when they include supervised resistance weight-training (or physical therapy for those in the bedridden setting) and controlled high-protein nutrition.

As can be discerned from this list of questions, we are far from answering the basic questions on the optimal use of anabolic steroids for HIV disease therapy. We invite physicians and researchers to join us in this effort.

Complementary Approaches to Treating Lipodystrophy

by Michael Mooney
(original version in
Medibolics 2(2), Nov. 1997)

While the protease inhibitor (PI) cocktails can bring viral loads down to undetectable levels and have given many HIV(+) people a new lease on life, protease inhibitors are not always benign drugs. As we approach year four of the triple-combo era, numerous problems have appeared among people who are on protease inhibitors. One of the most common of these side effects (and perhaps the least understood) is the protease belly or Crix belly phenomenon. Crix belly, so named because it was mostly observed among people being treated with Crixivan, is a condition most notably marked by the appearance of a large protruding potbelly. (At the same time this is happening some people report that they feel like they are losing muscle mass and fat, too, especially in the arms and legs.) Another sometimes concurrent but rare condition is the so-called buffalo hump, which is a fat pad that grows on the back of the neck that resembles what is seen in Cushing's syndrome. Women are also experiencing an increase in breast size as the breasts seem to gain fat (called lipoma), and many people are losing fat in their arms, legs, and cheeks while one or more of these other things are happening to them. Lipodystrophy is the medical term that has been given to this syndrome, but it can also simply be called bodyfat redistribution.

It now appears that lipodystrophy is not a side effect entirely specific to Crixivan, but may be seen with the usage of any of the available protease inhibitors, and has even been seen to a lesser degree in HIV(+) people before protease inhibitors were available. However, the various cocktails of powerful drugs being used today to combat the HIV virus seem to increase the severity of this syndrome over the simpler drug combos of a few years ago, although there is discussion that one of the older drugs, D4T (Zerit) may play a central role in the problem. And in some cases, the addition of the appetite stimulant Megace to the protease inhibitors seems to increase the potential for bodyfat redistribution.

There are several reasons why this might happen. Crix-belly in many respects resembles the potbelly seen in disease states like Cushing's syndrome, alcoholic hepatitis, and heart disease. In these diseases the potbelly is associated with the development of insulin resistance [1-3] and is primarily composed of enlarged fat deposits surrounding the visceral organs, like the stomach, and liver, under the abdominal muscle wall and ribs.[4] The potential for liver burden or toxicity induced by many of the common AIDS medications has been documented and the protease inhibitors are no exception to this rule. Elevated triglycerides, liver enzymes, and blood glucose and even diabetes have all been observed in patients on protease inhibitor therapy. All of these conditions are symptoms of diminished insulin sensitivity, and we are seeing that the protease inhibitors' effects on liver metabolism are inducing a state of insulin resistance in many people who are on protease inhibitor therapy. Complications of insulin resistance include hyperglycemia (high blood sugar), diabetes, and cardiovascular disease, and the FDA has documented over 80 cases of diabetes that appear to be associated with protease inhibitor therapy.

Indeed, from early 1998, numerous studies have documented an association between the use of protease inhibitors and measurements that indicate insulin resistance is present including data by Kathleen Mulligan, Ph.D. of San Francisco General Hospital, confirming that protease inhibitors can cause the blood chemistry changes that are typical of insulin resistance;[61] Dr. Ravi Walli of Ludwig-Maximilians Universitat Munchen in Germany reporting that peripheral insulin resistance is common in patients on protease inhibitors;[62] and Dr. Andrew Carr of St. Vincent's Hospital of Sydney, Australia, detailing his hypothesis of the cytoplasmic (cellular) retinoic acid-binding protein type I (CRABP-1) biochemistry involved in the liver dysfunction that may promote insulin resistance.[63] Additionally, some people who are using protease inhibitors are being found to have accelerated cardiovascular disease, which is also a common outcome of progressive insulin resistance.

A look at Harrison's Principles of Internal Medicine shows us that lipodystrophy can be associated with insulin resistance, and so we see that the components in this puzzle, lipodystrophy; elevated triglycerides, elevated blood glucose,

Insulin Resistance

Insulin is a hormone that turns on the transport mechanism that brings glucose (sugar energy) into cells to become glycogen. When the cells are resistant to insulin, transport is compromised, so the glucose that cannot be delivered remains in the blood, which results in elevated blood glucose (hyperglycemia). This can lead to increased insulin production by the pancreas as the body increases its effort to transport the glucose, so insulin levels in the blood can increase, too. Insulin is one of the factors that stimulate cholesterol production, so elevated cholesterol can be a direct result of chronically elevated insulin levels. Excess blood glucose can also lead to overproduction of fat molecules (triglycerides), as the glucose is converted to fat for storage.

When there is insulin resistance distribution of fat molecules in the body generally is dysfunctional. Fat may accumulate preferentially in areas containing the most hormonally responsive fat cells and blood flow, around the internal organs under the stomach muscles and ribs in the visceral cavity (visceral fat).[4] Other areas where there are lots of receptive fat cells with a rich blood supply are behind the neck (brown fat pad) and in women's breasts, and these areas can also be problematic in HIV-related bodyfat redistribution. Fat may also decrease in subcutaneous fat cells where there are less receptive fat cells with less blood supply,[87] as found in the skin of the arms, legs, and face. A classic example of insulin-resistance associated distribution of fat shows itself in the appearance of a person with a beer gut.

Chronic insulin resistance is associated with diabetes, a distended belly,[4 7 91] cardiovascular problems, increased risk of cancer,[88-90] and other health problems. Insulin resistance can occur because of liver toxic medications, genetic predisposition, alcoholism, and aging. Consuming too many calories and the intake of excessive amounts of carbohydrates, saturated fats or omega-6 fats (found in common vegetable oils like corn, safflower and sunflower oils) can promote it, too.[52 55 68-70 77] elevated insulin levels; diabetes; cardiovascular disease; and insulin resistance are all appearing.

While this chapter does not offer a cure for bodyfat redistribution as protease belly, buffalo hump, loss of facial fat, or lipoma, it offers tools that are documented to improve insulin sensitivity that may help people gain some control over this problem until medical science gains enough of an understanding to solve it.

Does Crixivan Lower Testosterone?

Several doctors I have spoken to have told me that they have seen that Crixivan can lower testosterone production, and low testosterone production is known to correlate with increased insulin resistance in men.[5]

In contrast, women exhibit insulin resistance when testosterone is elevated.[6] However, low testosterone does correlate with increased visceral fat in studies with HIV-negative women.[7] One study showed that about 50 percent of HIV(+) premenopausal women have low testosterone levels, which was associated with low body cell mass, and a tendency towards having fat mass that is above normal.[38]

It may be that normalizing a testosterone deficiency while being careful about keeping testosterone blood measurements no higher than mid-normal would be beneficial to HIV(+) women to improve nutrient partitioning away from fat tissue while lean tissue increases. This is an area that needs more investigation, as not enough has been done to study testosterone and wasting in HIV(+) women.

We also know that the antiretrovirals can cause muscle myopathy,[8] so it can be several things (including low testosterone production) that might add up to a loss of lean body mass, and an increase in visceral fat.

While this remains to be proven, one of the things that was presented by Dr. Gorbach from Tufts University when he reviewed their Nutrition for Life Cohort (600 HIV+ men during 254 days on protease inhibitor combos) at the Bethesda National Institutes of Health conference, was that although people tend to put weight back on with protease inhibitors, his data assert that they regain mostly fat, not lean tissue. Note: fat weight is *not* correlative with survival, but lean tissue is.[9] The loss of lean tissue and reciprocal gaining of fat so that total body weight stays the same, is typical of early stage wasting.[10 11] This increase in fat mass again suggests an impairment in glucose disposal and insulin sensitivity.

For those who have lipodystrophy, I would be concerned about any apparent muscle wasting and have the blood testosterone levels checked, including both free and total testosterone. If total testosterone is low, or in some cases, even mid-normal for men, because of the tendency for HIV(+) men to have decreased free testosterone levels, which correlates with a progressive decrease in CD4 T cells,[39] a doctor should consider beginning testosterone replacement therapy. We should also note that free testosterone measurements appear to be more correlative with lean body mass than total testosterone in wasting HIV(+) men[12] and women.[13]

Women and Testosterone

Studies show that HIV(+) women who are losing lean body mass may also need testosterone,[13] but the appropriate dosage of testosterone enanthate injections for women is usually much lower than the dosage for men, between 2.5 and 20 mg per week. This is something for a doctor to determine by taking blood tests, usually two to three days after the fourth weekly injection for a representative average level. A number of HIV(+) women are using testosterone creams that are compounded by a pharmacy like Women's International Pharmacy (1-800-279-5708). However, testosterone enanthate injections deliver a longer-lasting blood level of testosterone than the creams, which have a relatively short life span in the body. If a cream is used, it is usually applied in a dose of between 2 and 5 mg two times per day, while the injections are best given once per week, as studies show that testosterone blood levels generally decline to baseline within about 10 days after injection.[14]

As women are much more sensitive to side effects from testosterone, the physician should monitor a female closely for any virilizing side effects, which include oily skin, acne, peach fuzz, hair loss, and clitoral enlargement, and immediately lower the dose or cease the therapy if these kinds of symptoms start to occur.

Normal Testosterone Levels May Not Be Enough (Men Only)

I should also note that finding the correct testosterone dose for each individual is not always easy, as data from studies by researchers like Dr. Judith Rabkin suggest that being HIV(+) can mean that the normal range for testosterone measurements does not necessarily apply to men. In her study with HIV(+) hypogonadal men, Dr. Rabkin found that the dose of testosterone enanthate needed to be above 200 mg every two weeks, in order for good quality-of-life. The dosage she found to be effective was 400 mg every two weeks (which I suggest is best given as 200 mg per week for more consistent blood levels, less peak/trough effect, and reduced potential for side effects). At 400 mg given every two weeks the men's blood testosterone levels averaged about 1100 ng/dL one week after the fourth injection (on a scale where the normal range is 300 to 990 ng/dL). In private correspondence Dr. Rabkin said that she is not sure whether 300 mg every two weeks would yield a satisfactory result or whether the men would respond satisfactorily if their average levels only reached 800 ng/dL. She said that some men did receive benefit at about 700 ng/dL though.[15] Remember, the bottom of the normal scale was 300, so the normal scale didn't seem to apply well to these HIV(+) men.

Free Testosterone

We assert that men's apparent need for testosterone at higher than the standard replacement dose of 100 mg per week (for HIV-negative hypogonadal men) may be the result of hormonal resistance to testosterone. Hormonal resistance appears to happen with several hormones in HIV pathology. However, studies suggest that the need for higher testosterone doses is most likely caused by elevated sex-hormone binding globulins and lowered free testosterone, which is common in HIV.[39 42] When this is the case, total testosterone measurements do not adequately reflect the person's state of health.

Supplementing testosterone to bring free testosterone levels in the body into an optimal range may be beneficial to hypogonadal men in general, by improving the partitioning of nutrients more towards lean tissue and less toward fat tissue, especially visceral fat.[16] Significant data also suggests that appropriate testosterone supplementation can improve blood lipid chemistry to reduce the potential for cardiovascular disease in men who are deficient.[50]

Testosterone Patches or Creams

We have reports that application of the Testoderm TTS or Androderm testosterone patches directly on the buffalo hump appears to shrink it. If this works, testosterone creams or gels might work better as the dose of testosterone can be much greater than in a patch. While a study of adipocyte (fat cell) chemistry does provide a rationale as to why application through the skin might work, application of a cream would not be likely to work to reduce the belly because of the greater distance from the skin through the stomach muscles to the fat cells inside.

Anabolic Steroid Improves Insulin Sensitivity and Glucose Disposal

One study showed that the injectable anabolic steroid nandrolone decanoate (Deca Durabolin) improved glucose disposal and lowered insulin levels when administered at 300 mg per week, while it did not have any effect at 100 mg.[40] While this injectable beta esterified anabolic steroid may have a beneficial effect on insulin sensitivity another study found that it appears to enhance non-insulin-mediated glucose disposal.[80] This study and other studies state that oral 17 alpha alkylated anabolic steroids, such as oxymetholone (Anadrol-50), oxandrolone (Oxandrin) and stanozolol (Winstrol) promote insulin resistance because of their effect on liver metabolism.[44][58] This raises questions about using oral steroids when lipodystrophy is present.

The Paradoxical Effects of Oral Steroids

However, oral steroids can decrease triglycerides (fats) because of their effect of increasing post-heparin hepatic triglyceride lipase, which breaks down triglycerides. [57][59] For this reason oral steroids may help to decrease visceral fat, although they promote insulin resistance, and I have had reports of each of the oral steroids stanozolol, oxymetholone and oxandrolone reducing the protease belly in HIV(+) males. Indeed, data from a retrospective study of 700 patients recently released by Dr. Douglas Dieterich gave indication that the use of oral and injectable anabolic steroids may be effective in decreasing the potential for lipodystrophy-associated body habitus changes.[60] More study needs to be done to confirm this trend, though.

Human Growth Hormone (Serostim)

While the relative ineffectiveness of GH as a muscle-building anabolic hormone is detailed in later sections, GH does appear to have a role in reducing lipodystrophy because of its effect on lipid oxidation (fat burning), as was asserted by a poster presentation from Dr. Gabriel Torres of New York, that was presented at the XII International Conference on AIDS in Geneva.[56]

It should be noted that Dr. Torres said that while five patients had partial of total reduction of fat redistribution on 5 and 6 mg doses of GH, which I assert are overdoses for most people, four of the patients (80 percent) had either elevated glucose, elevated pancreatic enzymes, or carpal tunnel syndrome, so GH at these doses increased the potential for serious health problems. Elevated blood glucose can lead to diabetes and the problems that result including cardiovascular problems, eye damage, and neuropathy; elevated pancreatic enzymes can lead to pancreatitis; and carpal tunnel syndrome is quite painful and may require surgery.

I suggest that if Serostim GH is implemented, it should be considered that Serono's full vial dose is an overdose and this may be why 5 and 6 mg doses caused these problems. It is advisable to adjust the dose down for each individual, in an attempt to gain the benefit without increasing the problems. At this time I have reports of a reduction of protease belly and other types of lipodystrophy with doses as low as 1 mg per day and up to 3 mg per day with no side effects. I assert that lower daily doses are safer than higher doses administered every few days, and at a correct dose growth hormone can be an important part of the tools that address the underlying metabolic problem. While growth hormone will have a less powerful effect at a lower dose, at the proper individual dose there will still be a significant effect on fat cell metabolism with significantly less potential for side effects.

Exercise

Exercise, too, improves insulin sensitivity,[17] so people with insulin resistance should consider some kind of regular exercise, especially weight-training, which also builds lean body mass. Aerobic exercise does not build significant lean body mass. Aerobics may be useful in an effort to reduce lipodystrophy but if a person is losing lean body mass it should be avoided at least until the person has regained any lost weight or stabilized. Aerobics will use energy that the body would normally use for rebuilding lean body mass, only accelerating the loss of lean body mass. If your weight is stable and not in danger of losing weight, to optimally burn fat and reduce lipodystrophy I suggest doing aerobics three times per week on alternate days to weight training days, first thing in the morning on an empty stomach. (See the exercise chapter on page 129.)

Nutritional Considerations

Carbohydrates

I would also suggest altering your diet so that it is balanced somewhat like what might be called an "evolutionary-type hunter-gatherer diet." This means getting more protein and a moderate amount of the healthy types of fats, while eating fewer high-calorie, starchy, complex carbohydrates or high-glycemic, sugary, simple carbohydrates.

Currently, many progressive nutritionists are recommending that people with insulin resistance consider reducing their total calorie intake and intake of high-calorie complex carbohydrates that can release into the blood stream quickly,[18] including wheat breads and most processed wheat products. These kinds of carbohydrates actually are quite calorie dense and can upset insulin metabolism as much as sweets.[19][20] They are even more problematic when included in high fat foods. (Think pizza and ice cream.) Also on the list of carbohydrates to avoid is the sugar called fructose, which is known to promote insulin resistance, and raise cholesterol.[51] Look for it on ingredient panels as fructose or high-fructose corn syrup. I also underline that some people will experience a reduction in insulin resistance just by reducing the total calories in their diet, as many people simply eat too many calories. *However, if you are having a hard time maintaining weight because of wasting or infection, getting plenty of healthy calories is essential for keeping and building lean body mass, so be careful about reducing your intake of food.*

At the same time, I recommend an increase in the intake of complex carbohydrates sources that contain less total calories but lots of fluid and nutrients, like vegetables. Compared to grains, vegetables are more nutrient dense, and less calorie dense. While some vegetables like potatoes and carrots have high glycemic indexes, they supply good amounts of nutrients per calorie, and they do not contain a great amount of calories for their volume like grains or sweets do, so their effect on insulin produc-tion, insulin resistance and bodyfat accumulation is not as great. (Carrots contain only 195 calories per pound, boiled potatoes contain 450 calories per pound, while breads contain about 1200 to 1500 calories per pound, and sugar and sweets contain about 1700 calories per pound.)

Other good carbohydrate sources are beans, yams and green peas, and whole fruits like oranges, grapes, apples, pears, and cherries. In other words try to eat natural food carbohydrate sources that are one step away from nature.

If you do want to include grains in your diet, barley, cream of rye, oatmeal and brown rice have relatively lower glycemic indexes than most wheat products, but be careful to moderate the total amount of these high calorie starch sources. If you include them in your diet, I suggest eating servings that are about one third as much you'd really like to eat. (Again, try to moderate your total carbohydrate calories if your goal is to reduce insulin resistance.)

While a high-carbohydrate diet has been recommended by some nutritionists for conditions of insulin resistance (diabetes), a study by Chen of Stanford University, showed that a lower-fat, higher-carbohydrate diet led to higher day-long blood glucose, insulin, and triglycerides, as well as post-prandial (after a meal) accumulation of triglycerides, and increased VLDLs (very low density lipoproteins),[55] which can increase the risk of cardiovascular disease. The idea that lower carbohydrates diets are superior is supported in an article in Nutrition Reviews by dietitian Nancy Sheard, who said, *"Recent studies indicate that a diet high in monounsaturated fat and low in carbohydrate can produce a more desirable plasma glucose, lipid, and insulin profile."*[77] A study published in the Journal of the American Medical Association further supported this approach when it showed significantly elevated triglycerides and LDL cholesterol levels with a high carbohydrate diet, while a high-monounsaturated fat diet let to a lower-risk lipid profile.[78]

Fats

While it is also best to reduce any excessive intake of fats, I don't advocate a very low-fat diet, but a reduction in excess saturated fats, found in animal fat products like butter and lard, and excess omega-6 fats, which are found in common vegetable oils, like corn, safflower, and sunflower oils. Excess saturated fats and omega-6 fats can promote insulin resistance.[52][68-70] At the same time I recommend a moderate intake of fresh food sources of the essential fatty acid called omega-3, which can reduce insulin resistance,[52] and reduce the potential for atherosclerosis and heart attacks.[65][66] Omega-3 fats are found abundantly in cold water fish like salmon, sardines, tuna, rainbow trout, anchovies, and herring, and in lesser amounts in flax seed oil, some nuts and seeds and beans, like walnuts, pumpkin seeds and soy beans, and in much smaller quantities in dark green leafy vegetables. Consider also including some daily consumption of monounsaturated fats from sources like olive oil. These too reduce the risk of cardiovascular disease.

Data also suggests that high saturated fat in the diet promotes more bodyfat accumulation compared to polyunsaturated fats like omega-3 fats,[85][86] so if you want to be lean, eat clean.

Finally, avoid eating any food that contain artificial fats or processed fats, like hydrogenated or partially hydrogenated oils. Partially hydrogenated oils are found in foods like margarine, french fries, potato chips, shortening, many baked goods, and mayonaise. Harvard researchers have found a very strong link between these types of unhealthy fats and cardiovascular disease.[79]

Protein

HIV has protein malnutrition as a common theme; a lack of optimal protein contributes to the loss of lean body mass and trouble maintaining it. To reduce the loss of lean body mass and to increase it, I suggest that your diet include extra protein that totals at least 3/4 gram per pound of body weight per day. If you lift weights, studies by world-renowned protein scientist Dr. Peter Lemon show that you may need a total of at least 0.8 grams of protein per pound of body weight per day for optimal increases in lean body mass.[71][72] If you are not allergic to dairy protein, consider eating cottage cheese as a "best" protein for building muscle, as it contains a great amount of the amino acid L-glutamine, which is discussed below. (Note: dairy allergy can cause diarhhea.)

Also consider supplementing your food protein with a protein powder drink two or three times per day. Note that the dairy protein called casein, seen on labels as calcium caseinate, appears to have the potential to be somewhat more effective for improving lean body mass than other proteins, like whey.[73]

The Zone Diet

Although I do not agree with some of his more dogmatic concepts, my recommendations for nutrition have some similarities to the "zone" diet outlined in the book *Mastering the Zone*, by Dr. Barry Sears. While aspects of the zone diet can be criticized scientifically, I have had numerous reports that the use of the zone diet has helped people with HIV reduce cholesterol, the potbelly, triglycerides, and lipodystrophy symptoms, in general.

The Atkins Diet

The Atkins diet is a very low carbohydrate, high protein, high fat diet that can decrease bodyfat significantly. I have reports of people successfully using the Atkins diet to reduce lipodystrophy symptoms. Consider that it is basically impossible to get the RDA of vitamins, minerals or fiber from this diet, so if you use it, take strong multi-vitamins and extra fiber, and consider that it shouldn't be used long-term. Also be sure to favor monounsaturated and omega-3 fats over omega-6 and saturated fats.

Dietary Supplements

Supplements that have been shown to improve insulin sensitivity include chromium,[21] and I recommend 200 to 400 micrograms (mcg) of chromium three times per day in the polynicotinate or picolinate form, as one recent (non-HIV) study showed that 1,000 mcg of chromium per day increased insulin sensitivity by about 40 percent without toxicity.[22]

The herb silymarin (milk thistle) as a standardized extract in a dose of 200 mg three times per day has been shown to be effective in improving liver function and improving insulin sensitivity.[41] There has been talk that silymarin can alter liver function in a way that might affect the metabolism of protease inhibitors, so it is possible that people who are taking protease inhibitors should not take silymarin. There is no conclusive data on this yet.

But the *best* supplement for improving insulin sensitivity and glucose disposal may be the antioxidant called alpha lipoic acid (ALA), at 100 to 300 mg three times per day.[23] ALA improves insulin dependent and non-insulin dependent glucose uptake, and it has been shown to effectively lower blood sugar comparable to insulin itself.[24] I believe this is one very important reason ALA is a must for anyone taking HIV medications, especially the protease inhibitors. HIV-nutrition expert Lark Lands, Ph.D., asserts that ALA is a must for people with HIV because of its effect on improving glutathione production and recycling.[25] Studies last year at Stanford University showed that glutathione levels directly correlate with increased survival for people with HIV.[26]

As noted by the late Canadian protein chemist Chester Myers, Ph.D., N-acetyl cysteine (NAC) can be a valuable addition to the supplements that address lipodystrophy, because of its effect on improving glutathione, which is necessary for glucose tolerance factor metabolism. I suggest 500 to 1,000 mg of NAC three times per day.

Also carnitine, as the prescription version called Carnitor, would be beneficial in higher doses, about 500 to 1,000 mg three times per day, as it helps to lower triglycerides,[27] which are generally elevated when lipodystrophy is present. Note that the acetyl-L-carnitine form of carnitine may be more effective than plain carnitine, but it is more expensive.

Also worth considering is the omega-3 dietary supplement called EPA (fish oil), which has been shown to reduce insulin resistance,[52] and lower triglycerides somewhat in a study with HIV(+) men.[28]

And taking a strong multivitamin, multimineral supplement that includes chromium, vitamins A, D, E and calcium and magnesium will help improve insulin sensitivity.[29-33] [67] I recommend taking a supplement that contains doses that are much higher than the RDAs, though, as numerous studies have shown that higher nutrient levels are required in HIV disease.[53] [54]

Finally, high dose biotin supplementation is frequently prescribed by nutritionally-oriented medical doctors to improve glucose metabolism in diabetes.[74] [75] High dose biotin is also known to improve diabetic neuropathy.[76] The dose of biotin that is commonly used is 1,000 mcg three times per day.

Cardiovascular Disease

As I mentioned in the beginning of this article, we are also beginning to see cardiovascular disease in people on protease inhibitors. When cardiovascular disease is a consideration, we want to make sure that specific preventive nutrients are included. While there are many that can be included for this purpose, to keep it simple I suggest the following: vitamin E at 400 to 800 IU three times per day to reduce the potential for oxidation of blood fats that can contribute to atherosclerosis;[46] vitamin C at 1,000 to 2,000 mg three times per day to assist vitamin E in reducing blood fat oxidation;[47] folic acid at 800 mcg three times per day to reduce the potential for elevated homocysteine, which appears to be another major contributory factor to cardiovascular disease.[43] [48] It should also be noted that vitamins B6 at 50 mg three times per day and vitamin B12 at 100 to 500 mcg three times per day help to reduce homocysteine. Of course, all HIV(+) people should consider taking high doses of supplemental B vitamins, as studies by Dr. Marianna Baum, of the University of Miami, showed that HIV-positive people frequently require 6 to 25 times the RDA of these essential nutrients to stay healthy.[53 54]

Glutamine

For any loss of muscle, Judy Shabert, M.D., M.P.H., R.D., asserts that supplementing with high doses of the amino acid L-glutamine, will help reduce the catabolic process of breaking down muscle tissue,[34] and a recent study of wasting HIV patients by Prang showed that this might be true. (See Dr. Shabert's article in the August 1997 issue of POZ magazine.) For frank wasting, HIV(+) people are using between 12 and 36 grams per day of L-glutamine. (One tablespoon is 12 grams.) I have friends who have halted their random diarrhea and improved their lean body mass using these kinds of L-glutamine doses, and in Prang's study wasting and diarrhea and were checked by using 30 to 40 grams of glutamine per day. Glutamine too, has been shown to have a powerful effect on improving glutathione production,[35] and glutamine improves insulin sensitivity.[83 84]

If you are losing weight I suggest that you supplement your diet with a tablespoon of L-glutamine added to each serving of supplemental protein two or three times per day between meals. If your weight is stable, L-glutamine may be supplemented at lower doses, such as one or more teaspoons per day.

(Important note: most dietary supplements only stay in the blood for a few hours, so it is wise to take them several times per day.)

Metformin

Realize that while taking dietary supplements, especially alpha lipoic acid, may help, it is wise to investigate the use of the drugs that are prescribed to improve insulin sensitivity. Ask your doctor about these drugs, which include metformin.[37] New data presented by Saint-Marc at the 6th Retrovirus Conference, in February, 1999 indicates that metformin may decrease visceral fat while decreasing blood glucose, insulin, and lipid levels.[60] Serostim can increase blood glucose, insulin and insulin resistance.[81 82] This means that metformin might be found to be superior to Serostim growth hormone because it not only addresses fat redistribution, but reduces some of the underlying metabolic problems that growth hormone can promote. An important consideration is that while Serostim is priced at $6,000 per month, which makes it inaccessible for a majority of people who have lipodystrophy, metformin is available with a doctor's prescription at any pharmacy, and if a person has to pay for it themselves, it only costs about $35 per month.

However, cautions about the use of metformin are warranted. Dr. Michael Dube, of the University of Southern California at Los Angeles says, *"Lactic acidosis is a rare side effect of metformin that is more likely to occur when there is some impairment of kidney function. Lactic acidosis, which can be fatal, is also a rare side effect of use of nucleoside analogs. There is no way to know at this time if using the two together might result in more frequent, or more severe lactic acidosis problems. In my opinion anyway, metformin and NRTI's therefore should only be used together with great caution. Also, keep in mind that metformin can lower vitamin B12 levels."*

I should also note that some people are finding that switching antivirals causes a marked reduction in some lipodystrophy symptoms. This is an area that is currently receiving a considerable amount of study.

My special thanks go to Jim Brockman, who was the first researcher in AIDS medicine to hypothesize that insulin resistance was involved in bodyfat redistribution. His guidance sparked my investigation into this important area.

Can Switching Anti-Retroviral Drugs Reduce Lipodystrophy?

by Nelson Vergel

While forms of lipodystrophy have appeared in HIV before the introduction of protease inhibitors (PIs), PIs appear to have a powerful effect on promoting new and unusual forms of lipodystrophy. This raises the question about whether lipodystrophy symptoms can be reduced if a person switches from PIs to other antiviral drugs.

Several studies have reported reduced blood lipids and glucose and/or reduced abdominal girth for those people who have switched from PI combinations to non-PI combinations that use Viramune[1] or Sustiva.[2] As shown below, a study by Martinez found that 23 people who switched from a Crixivan + Norvir, or Saquinavir + Norvir combinations to a combination that

---

Barcelona Viramune Study Results[1] (12 month update)

23 Subjects enrolled (11 women, 12 men)

Prior Regimens: Crixivan + 2 NRTIs = 18, Norvir plus two NRTIs = 2, Fortovase + 2 NRTIs = 1, Norvir+ Fortovase + 2 NRTIs = 2), Median 9 months of viral load suppression prior to switching (range 3-14 months)

New Regimen: Viramune (nevirapine) + 2 NRTIs

All 23 subjects tolerated Viramune. Twelve months after they switched to Viramune, their blood tests revealed significant decreases in the following:

Cholesterol - 30% average
Triglycerides - 62% average
Glucose - 21% average
Fasting Insulin Resistance Index (FIRI) - 45% average

Waist-to-Hip ratio: 0.91 reduced to 0.83 (subjects lost truncal fat). Twenty-two of the 23 subjects kept their viral load below 200 copies with a Viramune combination. CD4+ T-cell counts did not change significantly after switching.

---

included Viramune and two nucleoside analogs had their lipids, glucose, insulin resistance and waist-to-hip ratio decrease significantly after 12 months. 22 of 23 subjects kept a viral load under 200 copies after a year. Although lab measurements of altered metabolism and abdominal obesity clearly improved, twelve months after the switch none of the subjects' body shape returned entirely to its pre-PI shape.[1] Perhaps more time is needed for the fat redistribution to normalize. It is also possible that factors other than PI use affect body shape changes. It would be interesting to see how much exercise would improve the results of this study.

It is important to note that some people can not switch to non-PI combinations and have to use PIs if they have developed resistance to most nucleoside and non-nucleoside drugs. However, many people can switch from PIs successfully while keeping their viral load undetectable.

At the First International Workshop on Adverse Drug Reactions and Lipodystrophy in HIV in San Diego, June 27, 1999, Graham Moyle reported that 11 subjects reported improvements in bodyfat redistribution after they were switched from a PI to Sustiva (efavirenz).[2]

Another potential option is the new protease inhibitor Amprenavir (agenerase). Glaxo-Welcome, the maker of this drug, report that Amprenavir does not produce the lipid and glucose disturbances or incidence of bodyfat redistribution seen with other PIs.

It is too early to tell whether these claims about Viramune, Sustiva, or Amprenavir are going to be reflected in the real world, however, some physicians are already opting to prescribe them preferentially to people who are newly diagnosed with HIV in the hope that there will be reduced incidence of lipodystrophy.

Testosterone and Anabolic Steroids: Adverse Effects, Rumors and Reality

By Michael Mooney

There is considerable misunderstanding on the part of the public and the medical community regarding the true potential for adverse effects that may occur as a result of the use of testosterone and anabolic steroids. This holds true both for legitimate medical reasons at appropriate conservative doses and for non-medical (cosmetic or athletic) uses at high doses. I assert that analysis of all of the available data will yield a more balanced perspective that will position anabolic steroids as being clearly less dangerous than most of the medications that are commonly used for HIV therapy, including protease inhibitors, antiretrovirals, antifungals, and many other drugs. I have heard doctors and other people express concern that anabolic steroids can cause cardiovascular problems, cancer, prostate problems, immune suppression, Kaposi's Sarcoma, lymphoma, and other health problems. Some cautions are warranted, but the potential for these health problems is sometimes exaggerated, and in some cases, non existent.

Indeed, none of the several dozen studies on anabolic steroids and HIV(+) subjects have documented a significant association with any specific health problem so far. And with thousands of HIV(+) subjects using anabolic steroids since 1982, anecdotal evidence suggests that if anabolic steroids used in medically appropriate doses are causing significant health problems they are somewhat rare. Also note that steroids may cause subtle problems like sleep apnea that have not yet been clearly documented in HIV(+) subjects, that may define themselves as time goes by.

While there are many questions about adverse effects, one of the most common areas of misunderstandings centers around the idea that all anabolic steroids increase the risk of cardiovascular disease. Certain steroids, like testosterone, nandrolone and oxymetholone have more potential to promote increased blood pressure, which will promote cardiovascular problems if not effectively addressed. However, while many people assume that all steroids cause the blood lipid changes that promote cardiovascular disease there is a considerable difference in the minimal effect on lipids that can be caused by oil-based injectable beta-esterified steroids like testosterone enanthate and testosterone cypionate, the generally non-existent or small effect caused by nandrolone, another beta-esterified steroid, and the pronounced effect caused by the oral 17-alpha alkylated steroids. Oral steroids have been noted to have profound effects on lipids, seen as elevated LDL cholesterol, and decreased HDL cholesterol that may increase cardiovascular risk, where nandrolone has much less effect and testosterone has little, if any, significant effect.[1-4] This is why injectable steroids appear to be a wiser choice if cardiovascular risk is to be reduced.

In fact, good data suggests that appropriate testosterone replacement might reduce the risk of cardiovascular disease. For instance, clinical studies with elderly and hypogonadal men have shown a beneficial effect on blood lipids with testosterone replacement.[5] Recommended reading on this subject include two books by German physician Jens Moller: *Testosterone Treatment of Cardiovascular Disease — Principle and Clinical Experience* (out of print), and *Cholesterol — Interactions with Testosterone and Cortisol in Cardiovascular Diseases* (ISBN 3-0540-17097-9). Both are Springer-Verlag publications.

Other misunderstandings are related to the idea that testosterone replacement therapy might raise prostate specific antigens (PSAs) or cause prostate cancer. While there is one case study that states that testosterone replacement increased PSA secretion in one man,[6] other larger studies assert that there is no significant effect on PSAs with appropriate testosterone replacement.[7 8] And, while some studies show no association between testosterone and prostrate cancer risk, other studies assert that higher testosterone levels correlate with an increased risk of prostate cancer.[9] Note that low serum testosterone too, has been described as resulting in a poorer prognosis in advanced prostate cancer.[10] (It may be that too much testosterone increases progression of prostate cancer, but too little testosterone does, too.) Still, while most data show a distinct association between testosterone and tumor growth, a study of 100 prostate cancer patients showed no association between free testosterone, total testosterone, and tumor volume.[11] Other data supports the idea that estrogen dominance has a significant effect on prostate growth, especially with advancing age where testosterone declines relative to estrogen,[13 14] therefore inhibition of estrogen may be beneficial. This is definitely a complex issue that requires more controlled clinical data to resolve, but prudence dictates that if testosterone replacement is found to be necessary, the lowest effective dose should be used,

and any individual with a potential for risk should be followed closely, including monitoring PSA.

The potential for liver toxicity is another misunderstanding that is common with anabolic steroids. Specifically, injectable beta-esterified (oil-based) steroids are not toxic to the liver, while oral 17-alpha alkylated (17AA) steroids present some toxicity to the liver in a dose-dependent manner.[15 16]

However, the potential for acute liver toxicity with 17AA steroids appears to be considerably less than many other medications, with potential problems related to hepatic toxicity, including cholestatic jaundice with short-term use, and with long-term use there have been rare reports of peliosis hepatitis and benign and malignant neoplasms (tumors).[17-20] To be clear, as detailed by Zimmerman of Georgetown University, 17AA anabolic steroid-induced cholestatic jaundice usually manifests as "bland" cholestatis rather than the more potentially lethal inflammatory cholestasis. In general, neoplasms have occurred only with very high-dose 17AA steroid use ($\geq$ 100mg/day) over periods of 2 to 4 years, with 11 years as the longest recorded use that resulted in carcinoma.

These side effects are dose and duration dependent, and are two of the reasons that we recommend that the use of oral 17AA steroids be limited to 12-week cycles or the shortest amount of time that is necessary to gain the desired weight. For a reprint of Zimmerman's essay titled Hepatic Effects Associated With the Clinical Use of 17A-Alkylated Anabolic-Androgenic Steroids, email a request to access@access-medical.com.

For a comprehensive review of the literature related to testosterone's benefits versus its potential for problems in HIV therapy, I suggest reading a paper by Dr. Judith Rabkin titled *Testosterone Treatment of Clinical Hypogonadism in Patients with HIV/AIDS*, published in the International Journal of Sexually Transmitted Diseases and AIDS.[12]

Anabolic Hormones — Adverse Effects and Remedies

By Michael Mooney and Nelson Vergel

Anabolic steroids are medications with good risk-to-benefit ratios, but they do have the potential to cause side effects, *and each of them can produce side effects when the dosage is high enough.* Some steroids are less likely to cause problems though, especially when used in their correct dosage window. This is a brief look at possible side effects, with a list of the remedies that might help. *Use the prescription items listed below only when monitored by a doctor, as several of them, like Accutane, can be dangerous.*

Problem	Solution and Comments
Acne/oily skin — Caused by testosterone and oxymetholone, less by nandrolone, generally not by oxandrolone or stanozolol in men. Women are more sensitive and may have problems from oxandrolone and stanozolol, too.	*Accutane* — a powerful prescription item — 40 mg/day for one week sometimes stops acne if started at the first sign or as directed by your doctor. Some acne-like eruptions could be caused by fungi. For these cases, the use of Sporanox is effective. Some doctors also prescribe antibiotics, like tetracycline for acne with good results. Anti-bacterial soaps. Use a scrubbing brush and wash twice a day, especially after sweating during a workout. UV light or sunlight.
Hair loss — Caused by too much testosterone, and by oxymetholone. Rarely seen with nandrolone, oxandrolone or stanozolol, but they may cause problems for women.	*Proxiphen* prescription salve and *NANO* shampoo and *NANO* conditioner by Dr. Peter Proctor — phone (713) 960-1616. *Nizoral shampoo* — Available by prescription. *Rogaine* — Available over the counter. *Propecia (finesteride)* — Available by prescription. A few males experience decreased erections with finesteride, though.

Problem	Solution and Comments
Increased sex drive — Caused by testosterone and oxymetholone more than other steroids.	A problem? Sex drive can drop to nothing in HIV. Sex drive is part of quality of life. This is not necessarily a bad side-effect.
Impotence during a steroid cycle – Rarely caused by testosterone, or oxymetholone much more by other steroids. This happens more with other steroids because they do not support healthy sexual function. That is why we generally recommend that steroid cycles be built on a testosterone foundation.	*Viagra* — Available by prescription; enables robust erections. Ask you doctor about potential side effects. *Yohimbine* — Available by prescription; increases sex organ sensitivity. Can increase blood pressure. *Muse* — Available by prescription; inserts into the penis to enable erections. *Caverject* — Available by prescription; an injection into the penis that produces an erection that can last 1 to 2 hours. *Papaverine* — An older injectable medication, less expensive than Caverject. *Wellbutrin* — Prescription at 300 to 450 mg/day; increases dopamine. Anti-depressant. *Human Chorionic Gonadatropin* — First dose is 5,000 IU, then taken again one week later. Note: If impotence happens while on testosterone, try varying the doses of testosterone. E.g. Higher and lower.
Insomnia — Usually this is caused by dosages that are too high. Find the least amount that gives you a good result.	*Sleeping medications*, eg. *Ambien*. *Melatonin* — 1 to 3 mg, 1 to 2 hours before bedtime Avoid working out too close to bedtime. Limit caffeine, especially after 3 pm. Do not administer oral steroids after 6 pm.
Testicular atrophy – Caused by all steroids.	*HCG* – One 5,000 unit injection per week for 2 weeks, every 2 or 3 months.
Enhanced assertiveness – mostly testosterone, and oxymetholone, but they can all increase drive, depending on dosage.	Great! HIV (+) individuals often have low energy, so this means wake up and live, or workout harder at the gym. Decrease caffeine. Meditation, yoga. The steroid dosage may be too high, especially testosterone and oxymetholone.
High blood pressure - testosterone, oxymetholone, nandrolone. Sometimes this is promoted by elevated hematocrit, and sometimes by steroid doses that are too high.	*Blood pressure medications* — Elevated blood pressure is usually transient and stops within a few weeks of the end of a steroid cycle. *Supplements* — Magnesium (600 mg/day); Vitamin B-6 (100 to 200 mg/day); may help reduce water retention. *Water* — Drink extra water every day to help flush the kidneys.

Problem	Solution and Comments
Gynecomastia (male breast development) — Caused by overproduction of estrogen, which can happen when is there is too much testosterone. (Testosterone converts into estrogen.) Oxymetholone may also cause it. Nandrolone is less likely to, while oxandrolone and stanozolol shouldn't. Growth hormone also seems to promote it. See the discussion below.	*Arimidex* - Inhibits estrogen production. Available by prescription. 1 mg/day until sensitivity stops, then 1/2 mg every other day. *Nolvadex* — Competes with estrogen for receptors. Available by prescription, 10 to 20 mg/day. Not as effective as Arimidex. Use of Nolvadex during a steroid cycle may reduce the net anabolic effect, as it decreases the production of GH[1] and IGF-1.
Virilization (body hair growth, deepened voice, clitoral growth in women) – Caused by testosterone, and oxymetholone, less by nandrolone, much less by stanozolol. Generally not by oxandrolone.	Discontinue steroid use or only use steroids that have the lowest androgenic potential, like oxandrolone. We note that GH used with steroids seems to exacerbate body hair growth in males. *Proscar* — Available by prescription.
Prostate enlargement — testosterone and oxymetholone. Nandrolone less. Oxandrolone and stanozolol have even less potential to cause this and may not have an effect at all. This is not clear.	*Proscar* - Available by prescription. For men, 1 to 5 mg/day. (Note: Can cause decreased sex drive in some men.) *Hytrin* - Available by prescription. *Saw palmetto extract* — Very effective for reducing prostate problems, but one study suggests that this herb may reduce the effects of testosterone, too.[9] *Estrogen inhibitors like Arimidex*. Estrogen dominance appears to increase prostate growth.[10][11] Check your prostate specific antigen (PSA) before starting any steroid program, to detect potential for prostate cancer, especially if you are over 35 or have a family history of prostate problems, and have it checked on a regular basis.
Polycythemia (Elevated hematocrit, which means there are too many red blood cells) — Caused by testosterone, nandrolone and oxymetholone, much more than oxandrolone or stanozolol. Crixivan appears to promote polycythemia.	*Therapeutic phlebotomy* means to have a pint or more of blood removed, usually 1 pint per week over several weeks. (1 pint usually will lower hematocrit by about 3 points.) Polycythemia is a compelling reason to avoid using higher steroid doses than are necessary. Taking the lowest effective dose reduces the risk of over-production of hemoglobin (red blood cells).

Problem	Solution and Comments
Elevated liver enzymes — Incidence is often exaggerated, but is related to 17-alpha alkylated oral steroids, not oil-based injectable steroids. Note: Injectable stanozolol, which is not approved for human sales in the U.S., is also 17-alpha alkylated.	**One or more of the following:** *Standardized silymarin (milk thistle herb)* - 160 mg/three times/day. *Evening primrose oil* — 1300 mg/three times/day. *Lung Tan Xie Gan* — Chinese herb formula. *Alpha lipoic acid* — 100 to 300 mg/three times/day. *Glycyrrhizinate Forte* - Three or more capsules/day. *N-acetyl cysteine* — 600 mg/three times/day. *Glutamine powder* — 4 to 12 grams/three times/day. *Omega-3 fatty acids* — 6 to 10 capsules/day. If there is a history of liver problems, avoid oral steroids and stay with the injectable steroids — testosterone or nandrolone. *Antioxidant vitamins* — Vitamin C - 1,000 to 2,000 mg/three times/day with vitamin E - 400 to 800 IU three times/day.

Anabolic Steroids and Kaposi's Sarcoma

by Nelson Vergel

Some physicians fear that implementing anabolic steroid therapy may induce Kaposi's sarcoma (KS) or increase its progression. KS has been found to be caused by a herpes-family virus. Although no controlled research has been performed on this, there are data that infer a relationship between hormones and KS. For instance, there is research showing that corticol steroids like prednisone can increase KS progression in HIV(+) patients.[1-3] (Note: Corticol steroids are *not* anabolic steroids, but they are sometimes confused with each other.) Some researchers hypothesize that, since most forms of KS are more common in men than women,[4] there must be a connection between male hormones and KS. Two notable papers on this topic were presented at the 1993 International AIDS Conference (Japan). One investigated whether hormonal factors contribute to a higher incidence of KS in men than women, and found no relationship.[5] The second paper found that men with KS had significantly higher levels of dehydroepiandrosterone (DHEA) and estradiol than those HIV(+) non-KS patients with the same CD4 levels.[6] When compared to non-KS patients, DHEA and testosterone were higher in patients with more than 500 CD4s; DHEA and testosterone were higher in patients with 200 to 500 CD4s, and DHEA was higher and testosterone lower in patients with less than 200 CD4s. It also found that estrogen and glucocorticoids were not significantly different in the two groups. Notably, this study found that the decrease in CD4 counts and progression to AIDS is accompanied by a decrease in serum testosterone. Unfortunately, other hormones in the hypothalamic-pituitary-gonadal axis, that may play a role here, such as leutinizing hormone (LH), and follicle stimulating hormone (FSH), were not measured in this study.

Another study done on men with CD4s below 132, which did measure total and free testosterone, estrogen, luteinizing and follicle stimulating hormones, found that *all patients with KS had lower testosterone and estrogen levels, and higher FSH than KS-free AIDS patients, AIDS-related complex patients, and asymptomatic HIV(+) individuals.*[7] A study performed in women found that low estrogen is common in females with KS, HIV(+) or not.[8] So, there appear to be confusing patterns with high/low testosterone or estrogen levels. It may be that another hormonal factor is involved, maybe something women's bodies produce that makes them less susceptible to KS than men. I think part of the answer to this question may be found in the studies that are looking at the beta form of human chorionic gonadotropin (b-HCG) as a treatment for KS. Women produce HCG during the early stages of pregnancy and it is extracted from their urine. One study showed that KS cells are killed in vitro and in vivo (apparently by apoptosis, programmed cell death) by b-HCG.[9] Dr. Robert Gallo observes that women's KS lesions subside during pregnancy.[10] He notes that b-HCG is similar to leutinizing hormone, which is produced at high levels during the menstrual cycle. This, he says, may account for the observation that KS occurs less in HIV(+) women than men. He does not point at men's higher testosterone as a culprit for this difference in incidence.

Many doctors have success injecting b-HCG in KS lesions. Notably, HCG increases men's testosterone production dramatically. So, HCG may help treat KS, but at the same time it increases testosterone. (This is another weak link in the theory that testosterone increases KS.) Dr. Marcus Conant (San Francisco), Dr. Parkesh Gill (USC-LA), Dr. Walter Jekot (Los Angeles), Dr. Patricia Salvato (Houston), and Dr. Gary Bucher (Chicago), assert that they haven't seen a higher KS incidence in patients being treated with anabolic steroids. Furthermore, Dr. Bucher concluded a 73-patient study using nandrolone decanoate. Eight of them had KS prior to the study. At conclusion no significant differences in KS were seen between the controls and participants. Dr. Bucher feels sure that there is no anabolic steroid/KS relationship.

The incidence of KS has dropped dramatically with the advent of protease inhibitors. I have seen dozens of people go into remission, once they start protease inhibitor therapy.

We welcome a clear resolution to this question through controlled studies, but at this time it appears that there is no direct relationship between testosterone and KS. Since KS is less common, this may not be as relevant as it once was.

Anabolic Steroids for AIDS Therapy: A Comparison Table

by Michael Mooney

The table on the next page is designed to clear up some of the misconceptions regarding anabolic steroids as therapeutic agents for AIDS-related wasting therapy. This table is a guide to weighing the relative risks to benefits for some of the common steroid analogs that are available in the United States and other countries. It merges anecdotal information from my survey of doctors and athletes over many years and the published data. Please note, all anabolic steroids can inhibit the body's production of its own testosterone; and all can produce side effects when the dose is high enough.

Note:

Five stars = highest rating; one star = lowest rating. Some good muscle-building steroids are given lower ratings because they may have more potential for side effects.

1. Nandrolone decanoate, a generic drug, should cost about $14.00 (California price) for a 200 mg bottle, whereas Deca Durabolin (trade name by Organon) costs about $25 to $35 for the same compound. Generic nandrolone was not available at press time, November, 1999.
2. Some studies show that specific anabolic steroids have beneficial effects on specific immune functions.[1,2,5,6,14] Differences in how specific anabolic steroids affect the immune system in HIV should be studied. Many HIV doctors prescribe testosterone and the other anabolic steroids and see improvements in critical components of the immune system, such as CD8 T cells.[14] Studies show that testosterone can delay the progression of immune diseases, like the autoimmune disease lupus.[7]
3. Common oral/tableted steroids are 17-alpha alkylated. This presents a burden to the liver that can cause an increase in liver-specific blood tests because they may be somewhat toxic to the liver in a dose-dependent manner. Injectable steroids, except injectable stanozolol (not sold in the U.S.), which is 17-alpha alkylated, do not cause any significant liver burden.[3,13] Injectable steroids are generally preferred over oral steroids for this reason. However, injectable steroids may appear to cause elevations in multi-purpose liver function tests (SGOT, SGPT, and LDH) during increased muscular stress or other stress in the body. Steroid-free athletes with high metabolic and muscular stress may show some elevation of some of these blood tests, too. Numerous other drugs also elevate these

Comparison of Anabolic Steroids

Steroid	Anabolic	Androgenic	Effects and Side Effects with Reported Effective Dosages
Testosterone Enanthate or Cypionate ✪✪✪✪✪ (injection) Required for most steroid cycles. Available in U.S. and other countries. Very inexpensive.	High	Medium to high	For HIV(+) men, 100-200 mg per week for mainte-nance, strong effect on libido, energy, appetite. Higher doses increase potential for water reten-tion, hair loss, acne, gynecomastia (breast growth). Women, 2.5-20 mg per week (chance of virilization).
Nandrolone Decanoate ✪✪✪✪✪ Trade name: Deca Durabolin (injection) Best steroid for men. Available in U.S. and other countries. Inexpensive.	High	Low to medium	Very good lean muscle growth. For men, 100-600 mg per week is relatively safe for three month anabolic cycles. The 12 week Satler men's HIV study used 600 mg per week. Can cause some water retention. May decrease libido if used without testosterone. For women 25 mg to 50 mg per week (chance of virilization).
Stanozolol ✪✪✪+ Trade name: Winstrol (oral) Available in U.S. and other countries. Good steroid for men. Can be used by women. Relatively inexpensive oral steroid. (80 cents per 2 mg tablet = 40 cents per mg)	Medium	Low	For men, 6-32 mg per day added to 100-200 mg per week of testosterone. For women, 4-18 mg per day, with slight chance of virilizing. No water retention, but watch liver enzymes. (See item 3.)
Stanozolol ✪✪✪+ Trade name: Winstrol (injection) Not available in the US. Included here because some HIV(+) people obtain from overseas and self-administer.	Medium	Low	For men, 50 mg 3 times per week. For women, 15 mg 3 times per week. No water retention, but watch liver enzymes as this water-based injectable steroid is 17-alpha alky-lated. Slight chance of virilizing for women.
Oxymetholone ✪✪✪+ Trade name: Anadrol-50 (oral) Available in the US and other countries. Strongest oral steroid. Least expensive oral steroid per mg. ($12 per 50 mg tablet = 24 cents per mg)	Very high	Medium to high	For men, 10-100 mg per day. Most powerful, least costly oral steroid for building muscle. Supports libido. Dose-related potential for hair loss, increased blood pressure, water retention, body hair growth, gynecomastia, etc. HIV study with males and females, at 150 mg per day for 30 wks showed no significant side effects, and 14 percent weight gain. Some women reportedly are using up to 25 mg per day without problems. May decrease liver glutathione production. Watch liver enzymes.
Oxandrolone ✪✪✪ Trade name: Oxandrin (oral) Good steroid for women and children. Some men get good results, some don't. Available in U.S. and other countries. Expensive. ($3.75 per 2.5 mg tablet = $1.50 per mg)	Low to medium	Very low	For women, 5-20 mg per day. For children, 1/10th mg per kg of bodyweight or 2.5 mg per day. Does not stunt growth in chil-dren. For men, 20 mg or more per day added to 100-200 mg per week of testosterone. Possible liver toxicity at doses above 20 mg per day for adults. May interact with the p450 3A4 liver enzymes that metabolize protease inhibitors.

blood tests. Liver test elevations usually reverse with cessation of the steroids. Anecdotal evidence from competitive bodybuilders who use steroids in high doses, and published data in the medical literature suggest that the incidence of liver toxicity from oral steroids is somewhat exaggerated and rarely creates severe problems *in healthy humans.* I suggest that physicians be particularly sensitive to the discrete liver readings bilirubin, GGT, and the liver isoenzyme of LDH. Data suggests that these may be more consistent indicators than the multipurpose liver tests, like SGOT and SGPT, when looking for potential liver problems related to anabolic steroids.[11][12] Of course, it is prudent to respond to all aberrant liver function tests when pharmacology is complicated with compounds like the standard AIDS medications.

4. Virilizing means masculinizing. This can mean increased body hair growth, a deeper voice, etc. in males and females. Women may find that they start to get oily skin and acne, grow dark peach fuzz or a mustache or other body hair, have itching of the clitoris followed by increasing clitoral size, or develop other male characteristics with continued administration of steroids that are somewhat androgenic. These problems sometimes reverse if the steroid dose is not too high and steroid use is stopped immediately when side effects are detected.

5. Anabolic refers to the growth of muscle and is desirable for wasting therapy. Optimal lean body mass is highly correlative with survival in AIDS.[4] While increased androgenic potential can mean more potential for side effects and virilizing, some androgenic potential is necessary for healthy metabolism as natural androgenic activity is necessary for libido, energy, and healthy brain chemistry. Generally speaking, the less androgenic a steroid is, the less side effects there will be. However, all anabolic steroids have some androgenic potential, and steroids that have very low androgenic potential also usually have less anabolic potential.

6. The upper dosage listed for women is usually for severe wasting only. Women's bodies do not tolerate anabolic steroids as well as men in general, so doctors agree that it is best to be conservative in the dosages, except in special circumstances where there is severe wasting. The steroids that are more androgenic, like testosterone, may not be problematic if the dosage is appropriately low. It is wise to consider starting at the lowest dosage possible when women use androgens/steroids.

Disclaimer: Dosages listed are based on a survey of the dosages used by medical doctors, and are not the author's suggestions. This information is for your doctor's evaluation and is not to be construed as information to be used for self-medication. If you self-medicate, you do so at your own risk, as no responsibility is implied or intended on the part of the author or the publisher. These dosages are somewhat conservative and only provide a reference range, actual patient needs are highly individual. The dosage ranges given in this table have been verified by medical doctors familiar with AIDS therapy to generally cause no significant side effects when used appropriately.[8-10]

Program for Wellness Restoration (PoWeR) Anabolic Hormone Guidelines

by Michael Mooney and Nelson Vergel

This document has been re-written several times over the last three years as new research becomes available. We update it approximately every six months, and publish new information in our newsletter Medibolics (subscription information is on page 140.) and on our web site.

Introduction

Testosterone and androgenic-anabolic steroids are rapidly becoming common therapies in the treatment of HIV disease for males and females who experience loss of lean body mass or hormonal deficiencies. These compounds have been used since the early 1980s by progressive doctors in Los Angeles for HIV wasting therapy and are now being used by many more doctors around the country. Dr. Walter Jekot, the first doctor to discover that androgenic-anabolic steroids were beneficial for AIDS therapy in the early 1980s, had patients who were using testosterone or anabolic steroids for cosmetic bodybuilding purposes when they came down with the new disease that was later to be called AIDS. Dr. Jekot noticed that his patients who used steroids maintained higher T-cell counts and suffered from fewer opportunistic infections than his patients who were not using steroids who progressed more rapidly and died. This is how Dr. Jekot discovered that anabolic steroids were beneficial for AIDS patients. After much initial skepticism, we found a number of inferences in the medical literature that support Dr. Jekot's contention that steroids, like testosterone and nandrolone may actually support healthy immune metabolism and improve long-term survival in HIV.[1-7] We have also interviewed some of Dr. Jekot's long-term patients and their statements support his position.

Recently released results of several controlled studies show the safety and efficacy of the use of these steroid hormones for HIV therapy. With the publication of these studies and the information that is available about the most effective methods for administration, there is little reason for HIV(+) people to experience wasting.

Our directive is to gather and refine information about anabolic hormones provided by doctors, the bodybuilding community, and HIV(+) individuals themselves, and share it with other HIV(+) people and their doctors. There are currently over 20 studies in the U.S. and around the world that are investigating anabolic hormone use. We have assisted some of these researchers to ensure that these studies include information already known by bodybuilders and the doctors who have worked with them. Anabolic steroids have been available since the 1950s and there is an abundance of non-HIV related information available to facilitate current research in this area. These documents summarize guidelines we have designed that are in use by clinicians across the country to treat HIV-related wasting and improve body composition for optimal health and longevity for HIV(+) individuals.

Rationale

There are several reasons for the administration of steroids:

1. When the person's body does not produce adequate amounts of testosterone or free testosterone the use of continuous testosterone replacement supports optimal physical and mental health and quality of life.
2. When a person has lost lean body mass, testosterone, combined with anabolic steroids promotes rapid gain in lean body mass. Use of this kind of combination is generally only necessary for a period of several months.
3. Maintaining lean body mass and a feeling of well-being over the long-term for some people requires testosterone replacement combined with a low dose of an additional anabolic steroid.
4. As part of a comprehensive program to address lipodystrophy.

Testosterone Replacement Therapy

Many male[47] and female[41] HIV(+) individuals do not have adequate testosterone function, primarily because the body's natural testosterone production is impaired, the amount of bioavailable testosterone is reduced, or there is inadequate expression of testosterone's effects at the cellular level. These may be complications of HIV-infection, but there may be other less well-known reasons for hormonal dysfunction, such as nutrient deficiencies that impair production of hormones or their reception and expression, e.g. zinc, vitamin A, and potassium deficiencies can decrease testosterone production or utilization.[114-116]

With progression of HIV, hormonal changes have significant correlations with immune function. Studies show that hypogonadism in HIV(+) people significantly correlates not only with loss of lean body mass,[41 47] but also decreasing T-cell count,[47] and increasing morbidity.[49] One recent study suggested that testosterone replacement therapy might decrease apoptosis (programmed T cell death) in HIV(+) hypogonadal males.[43]

In another study with HIV(+) men, DHEA and free testosterone levels decreased as CD4 T cells decreased in all patients.[48] In this study, low levels of free testosterone were common in all HIV and AIDS patients, and total testosterone and androstenedione were lower in those patients whose CD4 T cells were below 200.

For those who are deficient in testosterone, replacement therapy should be implemented using doses that are tailored for each individual. Once the appropriate dose is determined the person will generally experience improved quality-of-life, including better appetite, energy, improved mood, healthy libido, and immune function, and improvements in weight gain, functional strength and physical hardiness while suffering no significant side effects.

It appears that most HIV(+) people who need testosterone therapy will have to use it at replacement levels for the rest of their lives, or until a cure is found.

The Antidepressive Effect of Testosterone

We frequently hear HIV(+) people tell of how testosterone replacement therapy ended a long-time feeling of depression. One comparative study stated that testosterone replacement therapy produces equivalent effects to common antidepressive drugs (imipramine, fluoxetine, and sertraline) in the treatment of clinical depression in HIV(+) people.[44] While testosterone is not specifically defined as an antidepressive agent, restoring testosterone levels in hypogonadal patients can produce a powerful anti-depressive effect, possibly via its effects on neurological systems (dopamine),[94] and dramatically improve feelings of quality-of-life. Testosterone also has a very important effect on enhancing healthy libido for men *and* women.[80] [81] Dr. Judith Rabkin is now conducting a study to compare testosterone to Prozac.

Measurements

All HIV(+) people should be evaluated for testosterone function at HIV diagnosis and several times per year thereafter, first to see if they are producing enough testosterone, and then to see if they are responding optimally to the testosterone that their body manufactures by questioning them about energy, libido, mood, appetite, etc. Many HIV(+) people appear to be hormonally resistant to testosterone and do not respond adequately to what are considered to be normal blood levels of testosterone, so the doctor should consider that some people may require higher doses to experience testosterone's benefits.

Inadequate testosterone function means either that the person is documented to have low free testosterone blood levels, low total testosterone levels, or they do not respond normally to testosterone levels that measure in the normal range.

Hormonal resistance can express itself as low libido, low energy, decreased appetite, depression, decreased immune function, loss of body weight, decreased muscle tissue or functional strength.

It appears that a majority of male hypogonadism in HIV is caused by pituitary dysfunction, rather than testes problems.[47] To determine if the problem is in the brain or the testes, the physician should test for luteinizing hormone; if there is relatively normal or elevated luteinizing hormone coming from the brain, but low testosterone production coming from the testes, the problem is in the testes' ability to respond to luteinizing hormone. In HIV, testes problems can be caused by a number of factors including cytokine-induced inhibition of leydig cell function.

Hormone blood tests should be performed before any use of testosterone or steroid cycles. These include free and total testosterone for males and females to determine baseline measurements so that the doctor has complete information about the patient.

Elevated Hematocrit

Before any use of testosterone or anabolic steroids we also advise that the doctor measure hematocrit, as testosterone and anabolic steroids can increase hematocrit significantly, especially when higher anabolic doses are used. Thereafter, hematocrit should be monitored quarterly during any use of testosterone or anabolic steroids. We are also seeing an unusual increase in hematocrit when anabolic steroids are used with some of the protease inhibitors, especially Crixivan, so this may be an unusual effect of this combination that should be taken into consideration.

Some people will experience elevated hematocrit and hemoglobin with the use of testosterone injections, GH, or some anabolic steroids, which can increase the risk of strokes. If these are required for the person's quality of life and overall health we suggest that the physician consider that these elevations can be addressed by the administration of therapeutic phlebotomy (removal of one pint of blood) rather than interrupting the use of these hormones. Phlebotomy of one pint of blood will generally lower hematocrit by about 3 percent. We have seen phlebotomy given weekly for several weeks bring hematocrit from 56 percent to a healthy 46 percent. We know physicians who prescribe phlebotomy once every six weeks because of an unusual response to testosterone replacement therapy. This is a simple procedure done in a hospital blood draw facility that can reduce hematocrit, hemoglobin and blood iron immediately and easily in under one hour.

Prostate

A test for prostate specific antigen (PSA) should also be given to men over 35 years of age. While several studies show that testosterone replacement is not associated with elevated PSA,[119][120] questions remain about the use of testosterone replacement for men who have prostate cancer, and there are questions about the use of supraphysiologic (ultra high) doses of testosterone and anabolic steroids related to prostate growth. As noted before, compelling data suggest that estrogen dominance may be a primary influence, so this should also be considered.[140][141] Decreased progesterone has been cited as a possible factor, too.

Free Testosterone

While total testosterone is frequently the only measurement taken when hypogonadism is suspected, data strongly suggest that a free testosterone measurement is generally superior to total testosterone in evaluating testosterone function in both HIV(+) women and men.[93] For instance, free testosterone has been shown to be more correlative with optimal lean body mass than total testosterone in wasting HIV(+) men[42] and women.[41]

If the person has low free testosterone, they are a candidate for ongoing testosterone replacement therapy, whether or not they measure as having normal total testosterone. Sex-hormone binding globulin levels appear to increase throughout the course of HIV disease, and this progressively reduces the amount of free testosterone.[48]

It is important to do hormone testing in the morning on an empty stomach, as many things can affect free testosterone measurements, including diet. Elevated insulin caused by eating carbohydrates, for instance, can increase free testosterone levels by reducing plasma levels of sex-hormone binding globulin.[71]

According to the Merck Manual, normal free testosterone measurements for men generally range between 3.06 and 24 ng per dL. Optimal free testosterone levels for men appear to be in the midrange or higher end of this scale. For women the range is generally between .09 to 1.28 ng per dL. Optimal free testosterone for women appears to be in the midrange of this scale.

Also consider that inadequate response to normal levels of free testosterone can be the result of marginal or frank nutritional deficiencies caused by inadequate nutrient intake or impaired nutrient absorption caused by gastrointestinal problems, like diarrhea. Optimizing nutrient intake by using dietary supplements and improving gastrointestinal health by eradicating any detected parasites will often elicit improved sensitivity to the body's own testosterone or supplemental testosterone. Optimal response means that lower doses of supplemental testosterone produce better results with less potential for side effects.

Other Hormones

We also suggest measuring DHEA, GH, IGF-1 and thyroid hormone for men and women, and estradiol, and progesterone for women. These tests can be done by blood tests or by using the easy do-it-at-home mail order saliva hormone tests that are available without a prescription. Mail-order saliva tests for testosterone, DHEA, estradiol, cortisol and progesterone are offered by Great Smokies Laboratory at 1-800-522-4762.

Bioelectrical Impedance Analysis (BIA)

BIA should be instituted when a person is diagnosed with HIV, and measurements should be taken every three to six months if they appear to be weight stable. Doctors should perform monthly BIA tests during the use of anabolic hormone cycles to ascertain the effectiveness of the steroids.

BIA can be valuable between steroid cycles, so that if the person begins to lose over 20 percent of the lean body mass that was gained during the steroid cycle, steps can be taken to obviate further loss.

Liver Function Tests

For HIV(+) people who have extremely compromised liver functions, and because many of the AIDS medications have liver toxic effects, physicians should carefully monitor liver function tests when oral steroids are used. These include standard multi-function tests such as SGOT, SGPT, and LDH, and the discreet liver tests GGT, bilirubin, and the liver isoenzyme of LDH. One recent study asserts that GGT may be a more accurate indicator of steroid-induced liver problems than SGOT or SGPT.[45]

Types of Testosterone Replacement

Males and females who are hypogonadal should be given continuous testosterone replacement therapy in one of three ways:
1. Prescription testosterone injections;
2. As a prescription transdermal testosterone cream or gel;
3. Prescription testosterone patch (men).

Testosterone Injections

Injections are the most common type of replacement used by men, and are given at a weekly dose of about 100 to 200 mg per week if testosterone is supplemented in its most common long-acting injectable forms, testosterone enanthate or testosterone cypionate. For women the dose range is from 2.5 to 20 mg per week.

Injections have the advantage of once-per-week administration. Additionally, higher doses can be given to those men who appear to require higher blood levels, a common problem in highly progressed HIV(+) men. However, injections produce an unnaturally high blood testosterone level during the first few days after injection. Then the blood level drops off each day and falls to baseline in about ten days. (See the chart on page 74.) This doesn't effectively deliver normal blood levels of testosterone or mimic the natural daily pattern of testosterone release as well as gels, patches or creams can.

Additionally, if we consider testosterone's effect as a stimulant of red blood cell production, injections produce unusually strong stimulation during the first day and for a few days thereafter. This appears to increase the potential for elevated hemoglobin (too many red blood cells), and hematocrit. Creams, gels and patches appear to have less potential to produce this side effect.

Anecdotally, we hear that injections promote elevations in blood pressure more than creams, gel, and patches. It also appears that the effect on brain chemistry and the nervous system that might promote aggressive behavior can be stronger with injections.

However, some HIV(+) men do appear to need the higher level of overall metabolic stimulation that injectable testosterone provides; there is no one-size-fits-all approach that works for everyone.

We also find that a very small subset of HIV(+) men appear to need brief rest periods of 4 to 8 weeks with no testosterone injections because they become less sensitive to the effects of injectable testosterone after 6 to 12 months. This is something that a physician has to determine on a case-by-case basis by listening to the person's subjective feelings about their sexual function, energy, and overall feeling of well-being. If they report that they are no longer experiencing the benefits of testosterone therapy, and raising the dose has been tried to no avail, then they may be well served by taking a short 4 to 8 week break. Taking a break will usually help to return the person's sensitivity to the effects of testosterone injections.

However, we caution that people who really need to be on continuous replacement therapy can suffer a great loss of quality-of-life if they are taken off of testosterone, so the doctor should be sensitive to each person's evaluation of how they are feeling. If, a few weeks after the person breaks from replacement testosterone he or she is obviously tired, depressed, losing lean body mass, or feeling run down, it is probably time to begin administration of testosterone replacement therapy again. We see people for whom four weeks is enough break time, and others who seem to do well with eight weeks.

Testosterone Creams and Gels

We recommend considering the use of the testosterone creams and gels rather than injections for testosterone replacement therapy for both women and men. (Women generally prefer creams and men gels.) They appear to be considerably less idiosyncratic than injections because they produce more natural levels of testosterone without the high peak blood levels injections can cause.

Women's International Pharmacy recommends that creams or gels be applied two times per day, first thing in the morning with a second dose applied twelve hours later. After a few weeks of twice daily application, a relatively steady state blood testosterone level is generally attained, according to pharmacist Kathy Lammers. Some doctors prescribe once-a-day application of creams or gels and feel that this delivers a more natural effect. This application also occurs first thing in the morning to mimic the body's normal early morning rise in testosterone. Application to areas of the skin that have a layer of fat under them will slow the release of the testosterone so that blood levels are maintained longer. It is also recommended that the sites of application around the body are rotated so that optimal absorption is maintained. The best application areas include the stomach, the neck, the inner thighs, and the breasts. Be aware that some people complain about dark hair growth where the cream or gel is applied, especially if one site is used over and over again without rotation.

We also recommend creams or gels over patches because the amount of testosterone they contain per dose can be much higher that the 4, 5, and 6 mg patches; as much as 90 mg per gram. Additionally, patches cost about four times as much, with alcohol-based gels costing as little as $17 per month.

There are varying qualities of creams and gels made by compounding pharmacies around the U.S, and some of the poorer quality products are gunky and flake off after they dry, so buy from a reputable pharmacy. The best gels are clear and basically disappear shortly after application. Most men prefer alcohol-based gels, which absorb through the skin better than water-based gels. Creams should not be greasy and should resemble good moisturizing creams.

Some good compounding pharmacies include Women's International Pharmacy (800-279-5708), and College Pharmacy (800-575-7776), but there are many others around the United States and the world.

Also watch for Androgel, a very high quality clear prepackaged prescription testosterone gel made by Unimed Pharmaceuticals that should be approved by the FDA in late 1999. Early data on Androgel asserts that it may provide superior blood levels and pharmacokinetics compared to compounded gels. We have seen samples of it and were very pleased that it is exceptionally clean, non-sticky, and odorless.

Testosterone Patches — Men

Use of a testosterone patch like Alza's Testoderm or Smith/Kline Beecham's Androderm, or Alza's Testoderm TTS patches may be considered for men who need basic testosterone replacement therapy. Like gels, patches can be used to provide a base amount of testosterone when an anabolic steroid is used for weight gain.

Long-term use of Alza's older scrotal patch, Testoderm, might increase hair loss or prostate problems for some men, as one study stated that it causes increases in dihydrotestosterone (DHT) that are proportionately greater than the increase in testosterone because of enhanced 5-alpha reductase activity in scrotal skin.[118]

ALZA's newer patch, the TTS version of Testoderm, can be placed on other parts of the body, like the chest and back. While the Androderm patch can also be placed on other parts of the body, some people like the Testoderm TTS patch better because its glue is lighter and does not irritate skin the way the Androderm glue can. Still others think the Androderm is preferable because it sticks better and they report that they have no significant problem if *"mineral oil or tea tree oil is used to clean the glue off."*

We do not recommend patches used without an additional anabolic steroid for those who are wasting or need to gain muscle, as a study detailed at the NIH Wasting Syndrome Conference, May 20, 1997, at Bethesda, Maryland, showed that they are not effective for treatment of HIV-related wasting — the doses of the patches are too low. However, many people report improvements in libido, energy, and feeling of well being.

Replacement Doses May Not Reverse Wasting

Doses of steroids used for rapid lean body mass increases are higher than a typical replacement dose of testosterone given for hypogonadism. Effective injectable testosterone replacement doses for HIV(+) men for maintenance are generally between 100 and 200 mg per week. Rarely, we have seen men who are highly progressed who appear to require as much as 400 mg per week to respond adequately, apparently because of hormonal insensitivity.

We agree with Dr. Jon Kaiser that sensitivity to many drugs including testosterone can be improved by optimal nutrient intake, gastrointestinal health, and optimal nutrient absorption, therefore making lower doses of replacement testosterone more effective. Using lower doses reduces the potential for side effects.

Recently a study by Coodley showed that there was no improvement in lean body mass in progressed men (less than 200 CD4 T cells) who had greater than 5 percent weight loss when they were given testosterone cypionate at 200 mg every two weeks for three months.[38] This supports our concern that a 100 mg per week standard testosterone replacement dose *may be too low to effect a significant improvement in lean body mass for some progressed HIV(+) men.* Consider that a testosterone replacement dose for hypogonadal HIV-negative men is generally about 100 mg per week. Data in the published medical literature confirms that 100 mg per week is not enough to create a significant anabolic (muscle-building) effect for HIV-negative men,[82] although it may be enough testosterone to give them feelings of normal quality-of-life.

Finding the Right Dose — Men

One problem an inexperienced doctor may encounter is finding the correct replacement dose to get the desired beneficial effects for HIV(+) patients. Within its therapeutic window testosterone's possible side effects are not as serious as many other medications, but the doctor will get the best results with the least potential for significant side effects if he or she is careful in finding the optimal dosage for each individual patient.

We suggest starting with 100 mg per week to see if the benefits of testosterone, including more energy and libido, and improved mood and appetite are experienced. If, after four weeks there is not enough improvement, increase the weekly dose by 50 mg and after four weeks ask the person how they have responded. We also see a few men who do well with only 50 or 75 mg per week, while 100 mg causes problems. When the dose is too high the first noticeable side effects are usually oily skin and acne or irritability. If these occur, reduce the dose a little until the correct dose is found. The physician should also monitor changes in free testosterone looking for correlations with their patient's reporting of his status.

The Normal Scale Does Not Seem to Apply to HIV(+) Men

We suggest that the physician focus on listening to the patient's reports of their status and free testosterone measurements because the standard normal range for total testosterone blood levels may be too low for HIV(+) men. In an article in the Body Positive newsletter (May 1994, p. 22) regarding testosterone replacement for hypogonadal HIV(+) men, progressive researcher Judith Rabkin, Ph.D., of New York City, stated that in her study *those who experience significant improvements in sexual functioning tend to have higher serum testosterone levels, usually between 1000 and 1900 ng per dL.* (Remember the normal scale for men is generally about 300 to 1000 ng per dL.) In private correspondence Dr. Rabkin stated that a few of the men in her study did respond at blood levels that were as low as 700 to 800 ng per dL. The important point is that normal is a relative term, especially as it relates to total testosterone measurements, and it generally does not apply well to HIV(+) men.

This was further supported in another study by Wagner and Rabkin that showed that HIV(+) men with clinical symptoms of testosterone deficiency who had testosterone levels that were not only in the normal range, but exceeded 500 ng/dl, responded to testosterone replacement therapy with significant improvements in libido (89%), mood (67%), energy (71%), and appetite (67%).[142]

We suggest that if the patient is not responding appropriately to testosterone doses that deliver a free testosterone level in the low and even mid-range of the normal scale, the physician should consider working with doses that deliver measurements that register in the high end and sometimes above the upper limit of the normal scale. Optimum dosing can be very individual and it is best to be open to experimentation to find the dose that gets the desired effects of improvement in lean body mass, functional strength, energy, mood, increased appetite, and sexual function.

Physicians might also consider that the normal scale may be an inadequate measurement for HIV(+) people in general, whether they are hypogonadal or not. Thus we suggest that the physician listen to the patient directly rather than relying solely on the standard testing mechanisms and scales when making a determination of whether to prescribe testosterone replacement therapy and what supplemental hormone dosage is optimal. For women, the physician should exert great care in finding the optimal dose without overdosing, as women are significantly more prone to side effects than men.

(See the section for women on page 77.)

Testosterone Replacement Combined with an Anabolic Steroid

There are also individuals who function better, with less depression, and more energy when they use testosterone replacement therapy combined with an anabolic steroid. For them injectable testosterone by itself produces less than optimal quality of life. For this use the anabolic steroid can be considered to be a metabolic stimulant with indirect anti-depressive potential, in some respects similar to the use of compounds like classic anti-depressive medications such as tricyclics, mono-amine oxidase inhibitors, and SSRI's (selective serotonin re-uptake inhibitors). A typical combination that produces this benefit is nandrolone decanoate added to testosterone, with the person complaining that testosterone alone makes them feel poorly, but when nandrolone is added they feel good. Nandrolone's effect on elevating dopamine is documented in the medical literature,[121-123] so it appears that this may be a valid treatment for patients who suffer from depression. We have seen this many times over several years, and suggest that the physician be sensitive to the patient's needs and consider this use.

Steroid Cycling for Muscle Growth

Rationale Behind Cycling Anabolic Steroids

This section details the cycling approach, which is used for rapid weight gain. Cycling anabolic steroids is the backbone of the most effective program for gaining lean muscle tissue quickly for all HIV(+) people who need to, but this is not in lieu of appropriate testosterone replacement. Even people who have normal healthy testosterone function should be given a replacement amount of testosterone as a hormone foundation when cycling nandrolone decanoate (Deca Durabolin), oxandrolone (Oxandrin), or stanozolol (Winstrol). The use of any of these steroids alone will cause a significant decrease in natural testosterone production and with it a decrease in the beneficial androgenic characteristics of testosterone that are required for optimal quality of life. This can result in decreased libido, energy, and appetite. Only oxymetholone (Anadrol) has enough androgenic potential to be used without testosterone, and generally speaking it should be used with caution when combined with testosterone, as combining these two powerful androgens appears to increase the incidence of side effects considerably.

During the cycle the person should do their best to eat high protein meals, get good rest, and exercise consistently to increase their lean body mass as quickly as possible to what is ascertained to be a healthy level. The total dose of testosterone and the anabolic steroid that is combined with it should be high enough to create an anabolic environment in the muscle tissue so that it responds optimally to the stimulation caused by exercise. The anabolic steroids are used to add anabolic potential to testosterone, without increasing the potential for the androgenic and estrogenic side effects that testosterone might cause if it was used by itself at higher than replacement doses.

12 Week Steroid Cycles

While some bodybuilding books detail complex anabolic steroid cycle patterns, most of the time the simplest cycles are the best. Effective cycles can employ constant low, medium, or high doses of one anabolic steroid or a combination of steroids, or the ramp pattern that is detailed below.

In the first examples of steroid cycles all the available steroids except oxymetholone are added to a replacement dose of testosterone.

1. Nandrolone at 100 to 200 mg per week added to 100 to 200 mg of testosterone per week;
2. Stanozolol at 4 mg to 8 mg three times per day added to 100 to 200 mg of testosterone per week;
3. Oxandrolone at 5 mg to 10 mg four times per day added to 100 to 200 mg of testosterone per week;
4. Oxymetholone at 12.5 mg to 50 mg two times per day.

While anabolic steroid cycles are usually added to replacement doses of testosterone enanthate or testosterone cypionate injections, testosterone can also be administered as a transdermal cream, gel, or patch. Examples:
1. Oxandrolone at 5 mg to 10 mg four times per day added to 50 mg of testosterone gel twice per day;
2. Stanozolol at 4 mg to 8 mg three times per day added to 50 mg of testosterone gel twice per day;

Oral steroids are most effective when taken in divided doses several times per day as they stay in the blood stream for only a few hours after ingestion.

Oral Steroids Increase Strength

Some doctors prescribe "stacking" cycles that combine an oral steroid with injectables, such as stanozolol combined with nandrolone and testosterone; or oxandrolone combined with nandrolone and testosterone. Another possible cycle is nandrolone combined with oxymetholone, with no testosterone, although some men do use these three combined.

Hypothetically speaking, the effect of stacking an oral steroid with injectables may improve the total effect on muscle gain because 17-alpha alkylated oral steroids improve synthesis of muscle cell creatine, which improves overall muscle strength, significantly more than injectables.[131] There is also a possibility that increased creatine enhances muscle cell anabolic activity, but this is not known conclusively.

Ramp Cycles

Another type of cycle that resembles a ramp is utilized in the anabolic steroid cycles detailed below, including the high dose PoWeR cycle. The ramp approach, after an initial gradually escalating low-dose acclimation, plateaus at high doses during the middle weeks of the cycle, and then de-escalates the dosage gradually until cessation of the cycle to taper off the steroids. The purpose of this pattern is to ease up to the higher doses over a period of weeks gradually — some people feel wired or jacked up if they begin a cycle with high doses of anabolic steroids. During the middle high dose period be aware that you might have a tendency to be overly aggressive, or snappy. Catch yourself if you do and stay cool. The dose reduction in the final weeks allows you to ease off the steroids gradually so that you don't have a feeling of "crashing."

Moderate and Higher-Dose Ramp Cycles

As the table that follows shows, the first suggested moderate-dose ramp cycle provides a base of 100 mg of replacement testosterone plus 100 mg of nandrolone decanoate for the first two weeks. The nandrolone dosage is increased from weeks three to nine to 200 mg per week, for a basic moderate dosage, or 300 to 400 mg for the person who still does not gain lean body mass adequately at 200 mg.

The higher dose cycle is similar to the moderate dose cycle, but uses even higher doses during the middle of the cycle.

If in early evaluation it has been determined that a hypogonadal patient requires 200 mg of testosterone as a replacement dose, we suggest that testosterone be given as a 200 mg dose rather than 100 mg during the steroid cycle.

Higher Dose PoWeR Cycle

For high lean body mass gains when you have lost a significant amount of weight from an unexpected infection we suggest implementing the PoWeR cycle, which is being administered by HIV doctors around the country. The PoWeR cycle is also useful for those who are severely underweight and want to develop and maintain a ready reserve of lean body mass. This can be extremely valuable if you experience an unexpected opportunistic infection with accompanying weight loss.

Joseph

Joseph, was HIV(+) for six years when a bout with pneumonia caused him to drop from his normal weight of 185 pounds to 150 pounds at 6'1" tall. To regain his weight he instituted a comprehensive high dose PoWeR cycle and then over a period of two years used lower dose steroid cycles to build himself up to 235 pounds, which is an athletic level of lean body mass.

Joseph liked camping and the outdoors, and white water rafting was his one of his favorite releases. During one whitewater rafting trip Joseph took a dip and ended up swallowing water. Later that night he began to experience the beginning of a severe infection of cryptosporidium parvum, a water-borne pathogen that lasted for over a month. During the crypto infection Joseph lost 50 lbs before stabilizing at 185 lbs. If he had weighed 185 lbs when he contracted the infection and lost 50 lbs, Dr. Donald Kotler's data suggest that Joseph might have had problems recovering or even surviving. Joseph thinks that anabolic steroids probably saved his life.

Joseph's story provides an argument for the institution of the PoWeR cycle to help an HIV(+) person build a reserve of quality lean body mass so that they have extra lean tissue to burn in case there is an unexpected illness.

It is important to note that wasting is generally a later stage condition that follows internal decline. Starting steroid therapy when early wasting is detected, which may occur before there is overt external wasting, may prevent or slow internal decline itself, and so the potential for the person to progress in HIV may be reduced considerably. There are also people who do not respond well enough to low and moderate dose cycles, and seem to require higher doses.

Nelson

Nelson Vergel, who had wasted to 140 lbs in 1994, began his anabolic steroid therapy with a PoWeR cycle and put on 35 pounds of lean body mass in four months. All of his AIDS-related complex symptoms disappeared with the weight gain. After 17 years of infection, Nelson currently weighs 196 pounds with only 7 percent body fat. Nelson stays on a maintenance program that consists of 100 mg of testosterone cypionate and 200 mg of nandrolone decanoate per week and has never had to use another PoWeR cycle. Most of the time his quality-of-life is excellent with tremendous productivity. His liver and kidney function are healthy and his PSA is low. His only problem is borderline high blood pressure, but he had this before using steroids.

PoWeR Ramp Cycle Table

The chart details what we suggest as a very high dose, highly effective anabolic steroid cycle that has the least potential for side effects. Options are given for the use of nandrolone, with a base amount of testosterone, at lower and higher doses. In the PoWeR cycle, if side effects like acne or irritability are experienced, it may help to reduce the highest dose of testosterone to only 100 or 200 mg, while increasing the nandrolone dosage to make up the total milligrams in the chart.

Maintaining LBM Between Cycles

For people who have healthy testosterone production, we suggest a minimum 16 week period of total abstinence from any anabolic steroid, including testosterone, before instituting another cycle unless you lose over 20 percent of the weight you gained during the steroid cycle. This gives the body time to resume natural testosterone production and reduces the potential for permanent inhibition of normal testosterone production.

It is essential that two critical components be maintained when the steroid cycle is ended to best maintain the lean body mass that was gained:

- First, the person should maintain consistent optimal protein intake, including eating meals with a high protein content and perhaps supplementing the diet with protein powder drinks. Remember that men who lift weights probably need a total of about 0.8 grams of protein per pound of body weight per day, according to Dr. Peter Lemon, of the University of Western Ontario.[107 108] We recommend 1 gram to provide a margin for error. (People with liver or kidney problems should consult their doctor before increasing protein intake.)
- Second, a consistent weight-training program should be maintained. (See our suggestions in the chapter on weight-training program on page 129.)

Over the last few years, numerous hypogonadal people who clearly do not have adequate testosterone function have asked about cycling on and off all steroids, *including* testosterone. The majority of the time it is not appropriate for them to cycle off of testosterone, as they will experience a loss of lean body mass, energy, and overall quality of life. If anabolic steroids are used in addition to replacement testosterone in cycles by these people, maintenance testosterone replacement therapy should continue when the cycle of additional anabolic steroids ends. While some people only have to use one PoWeR cycle to gain 30 or 40 pounds, they may need to institute another cycle at some time due to a bout with a catabolic illness that causes weight loss. Still some people only require replacement testosterone.

Cycling for People with Healthy Testosterone Function

There are also individuals who have healthy testosterone function yet have a medical reason to gain lean body mass. This might be because

Men's Ramp Cycles

Cycle	1 — Moderate	2 — Higher Dose	The PoWeR Cycle
Week	Nandrolone dosage (mg) with base of testosterone	Nandrolone dosage (mg) with base of testosterone	Testosterone enanthate or testosterone cypionate (T) combined with nandrolone decanoate (ND)
1	100 mg	100 mg	100 mg T
2	100 mg	100 mg	200 mg T + 100 mg ND
3	200 mg	200 mg	300 mg T + 200 mg ND
4	200 mg	200 mg	300 mg T + 200 mg ND
5,6,7	200 mg	300 or 400 mg	400 mg T + 300 mg ND
8	200 mg	300 or 400 mg	300 mg T + 300 mg ND
9	200 mg	200 mg	200 mg T + 200 mg ND
10	200 mg	200 mg	100 mg T + 200 mg ND
11	100 mg	100 mg	100 mg T
12	100 mg	100 mg	100 mg T
13			
14			
15	Institute refraction guidelines on page 75 to return the body's natural testosterone production.		

Moderate & higher dose cycles. These cycles address moderate weight loss. For some, #1 alone is effective enough to reach goal LBM. Others need #2 or #3. After the cycle, take a minimum 16-week break, monitoring every 4 weeks for LBM loss.

PoWeR cycle. For those who do not respond well enough to low or moderate dose cycles, or who have lost 10 percent of normal weight. Afterwards take a 16-week minimum break, monitoring every 4 weeks for LBM loss. After the cycle if you lose 20 percent of the LBM gained during the cycle consider two options: either begin another cycle or add a low dose of a steroid like nandrolone (100 mg per week), stanozolol (4 mg three times per day), or oxandrolone (5 mg four times per day) to ongoing testosterone replacement. For many people, testosterone replacement at 100 to 200 mg per week will be enough to maintain weight.

they are underweight to begin with, and increasing their lean body mass would contribute to their better overall physical and mental health, or because they have suffered from weight loss caused by a bout with an infection. These people do not need continuous testosterone replacement therapy after a steroid cycle ends.

Cycling is important for these people because cycling allows the body time to resume its normal testosterone production after the cycle is ended during the rest period. It also reduces long-term inhibition of the feedback loop that controls testosterone production in the body.

Dr. Shalender of UCLA told us that it took no longer than 16 weeks (four months) for healthy HIV-negative men to return to normal testosterone production after his 600 mg per week, 10-week testosterone enanthate study.[72] He also confirms that the return to normal took no more than six months for the healthy men in his male contraceptive study that employed 200 mg of testosterone enanthate per week for one year. While long-term, very high dose steroid or testosterone abuse could elicit a more negative result and take even longer to return to normal, and may even cause a permanent inhibition of testosterone production, Dr. Bhasin's statement suggests that the body will resume its natural testosterone production after the use of the medically sound and reasonable steroid doses we recommend. Whether HIV(+) men have less potential for a full return of normal testosterone production is not known, however.

Refraction Guidelines — Men

Helping the Body Return Testosterone Production To Normal Quickly

All steroids cause the body to turn down its own testosterone production shortly after you start using them and testosterone production does not return to normal immediately after you stop using them. Refraction refers to the period of time after the use of steroids when the body continues to produce less testosterone than normal. Without intervention with our refraction guidelines it can take 3 to 6 months to produce normal testosterone levels again. But with these guidelines we have seen testosterone productions return to full normal levels after as little as two weeks.

Testosterone and Immune Function

Returning the body's testosterone production to normal quickly is important for those men whose bodies can produce normal levels of testosterone. When testosterone is low there can be an imbalance in the normal testosterone-to-cortisol relationship that favors cortisol, an immunosuppressive, catabolic hormone, as the dominant hormone. Testosterone and cortisol, in some aspects, are counter-balancing hormones in their effects on the immune system and muscle tissue. Reduced testosterone can allow cortisol to depress immune function, and break down muscle tissue. Cortisol depresses T cell production and catabolizes muscle, while testosterone supports healthy T cell metabolism and builds muscle.

We sometimes see bodybuilders coming off steroid cycles contract infections (especially upper respiratory infections) because cortisol, as an immunosuppressive hormone, weakens certain critical immune functions. This is one reason that it is important to quickly restore testosterone levels after cessation of a cycle.

Remember, this refraction protocol is for men whose bodies can produce normal levels of testosterone. It is not for men who are clinically hypogonadal before the use of steroids. If you are truly hypogonadal you should stay on testosterone replacement when you come off the cycle.

The Refraction Guidelines Cocktail

These three medications complement each other.

HCG (human chorionic gonadotropin)

HCG mimics luteinizing hormone (LH), the natural hormone in your body that tells the testes to produce testosterone. If the testicles have atrophied (shrunken) during the steroid cycle, they will likely begin to enlarge and up-regulate their testosterone production significantly shortly after HCG therapy is instituted. HCG "jump-starts" the testes.

While we have heard it stated that HCG addresses testicular function rather than brain center control of leutinizing hormone (LH), one study showed that while HCG raised testosterone production, it also increased LH significantly.[52]

We note that HCG may have therapeutic benefits for Kaposi's Sarcoma[54] and HCG's beta unit has anti-HIV activity in vitro.[55]

Administration: HCG is a water-based injectable medication, rather than an oil-based medication like common injectable steroids, so small 29-gauge ultra-fine syringes can be used rather than the larger (more painful) 22-gauge needles required for steroid injections. Most men inject HCG into the top of the thigh while seated. Ask your doctor for instructions on how to inject. HCG dosing is either of two patterns: preferred is 5,000 IU once per week for four weeks; the other option is 2,000 IU every other day for fourteen injections. Some men experience bloating, moodiness, acne, or hair loss when they use the 5,000 IU pattern, but they find that the 2,000 IU pattern causes no problems. The 5,000 IU pattern is much more effective though in stimulating testosterone production for the majority of men.

HCG can also be used by itself during the middle of an anabolic steroid cycle to reverse testicular atrophy (shrunken testicles). This method employs an injection of 5,000 IU of HCG followed one week later by another 5,000 IU during the approximate midpoint of the cycle, or any time that the testes appear to have shrunken.

Arimidex (anastrozole)

Arimidex, an antiestrogen, reduces estrogen production by inhibiting the activity of aromatase, the enzyme that converts testosterone to estrogen. Since the hypothalamus senses estrogen as one of the primary barometers it uses to determine how much testosterone to produce,[51] the decrease in estrogen induced by Arimidex signals the hypothalamus to increase leutinizing hormone releasing hormone. This causes increased production of leutinizing hormone, which in turn stimulates the leydig cells in the testes to produce testosterone.

Arimidex is a good partner compound to be used when HCG is used, because HCG can also increase estrogen and the potential for estrogen-related side effects substantially. Arimidex inhibits this effect.

Administration: Arimidex is taken at 1 mg per day during the 56-day refraction protocol.

Caution: Arimidex should generally not be used at 1 mg per day for longer than is necessary, as estrogen is required for healthy brain chemistry and cardiovascular health, so long-term inhibition can cause health problems. Long-term use to reduce estrogen in men is typically at a lower dose, such as 1/2 tablet every other day, as determined by testing.

Clomid (clomiphene citrate)

Clomid, another type of antiestrogen, can have a pronounced effect on return of important quality-of-life functions like libido, and feelings of well-being.[53] Clomid increases luteinizing hormone and testosterone, but does not appear to down-regulate testicular leydig cell activity, because it blocks testicular estrogen receptors as an estrogen antagonist.[54]

We caution that some men may experience mood changes and feel more emotional when using Clomid. For them HCG and Arimidex can be used for the full 8 weeks without Clomid. This should still produce a full restoration of testicular function.

Administration: 50 mg of Clomid is taken two times per day starting on day 29, after HCG administration ceases.

Testing

At the end of 28 days we suggest testing free and total testosterone levels to accertain how well the person is responding to this protocol. We also suggest testing again at the end of this protocol in 60 days and again in 90 days.

Growth Hormone for Refraction

Low dose GH administration may increase the effectiveness of the refraction guidelines because GH has been shown to improve the response of leydig cells to leutinizing hormone.[79] This improves testosterone production. Our suggested dose for this use is 0.5 mg (1.5 IU) per day before bedtime during the refraction protocol.

Note: HCG/Arimidex/Clomid therapy is not a perfect way to re-institute normal testosterone production quickly, but it can work very well. We are currently researching improved alternatives to what we suggest here, which will be reported in our newsletter Medibolics as we learn more. If any physician has feedback on the use of these refraction guidelines or suggestions for other methods, please contact us at (310) 360-0654 or email us at mmooney@icnt.net.

Women

Hormone Replacement Therapy (HRT)

At the NIH Wasting Conference in Bethesda, Maryland, on May 20, 1997, Dr. Donald Kotler explained that gender is correlative with differences in changes in body composition in wasting. Women tend to lose fat sooner than men in the process of wasting, and also regain fat quickly after recovery from opportunistic infections, and this is logically a result of differences in hormone levels in men and women; since men have higher testosterone levels and lower estrogen levels than women, it is easier for men to maintain more lean muscle mass with lower body fat.

We suggest that a complete hormone replacement therapy (HRT) program monitored by a knowledgeable doctor should be considered for all women living with HIV, especially if lean tissue loss is detected by calipers or BIA, if hormone analysis (saliva or blood) shows that hormone levels are inadequate, or if you experience irregular menstrual cycles or lack of menstruation, a symptom of hormonal deficiency. While in the past HRT addressed only estrogen, optimal HRT for women with HIV should take into consideration estradiol, progesterone, DHEA, testosterone, and thyroid, as each of these interdependent hormones can have a role in maintaining lean body mass and overall health. E.g. decreasing DHEA levels are associated with decreasing free testosterone levels and decreasing lean body mass in late-stage HIV(+) women.[41] Replacement doses of DHEA will also provide a significant increase in testosterone in women (but not in men[130]) so that testosterone replacement is sometimes not necessary. See also the section on DHEA that follows.

Employing complete HRT becomes more compelling when we see that one study suggests that HRT as estrogen alone may increase the risk of death in HIV(+) women.[101] While this informa-

Refraction Guidelines							
Week 1	**2**	**3**	**4**	**5**	**6**	**7**	**8**
HCG(see above)	HCG	HCG	HCG	Clomid 100 mg/d	Clomid 100 mg/d	Clomid 100 mg/d	Clomid 100 mg/d
Arimidex 1 mg/day	Arimidex 1 mg/day	Arimidex 1 mg/day	Arimidex 1 mg/day	Arimidex 1 mg/day	Arimidex 1 mg/day	Arimidex 1 mg/day	Arimidex 1 mg/day

tion has not been investigated in depth, physicians should consider that HIV disease progression may be increased by hormonal imbalance — too little of some hormones (testosterone, DHEA, and progesterone) relative to too much estrogen may create what amounts to a pro-inflammatory metabolism. It is known that in women a deficiency of testosterone, or an imbalance between testosterone and estrogen with relatively too much estrogen may increase progression of other immune pathologies, like the autoimmune disease lupus.[5] HIV likely has a similar potential.

After hormone testing is completed to ascertain replacement strategies, compounding pharmacies like Women's International Pharmacy (800-279-5708) can create whatever transdermal HRT cream formula is required for each individual. Call them to get an information packet that you can share with your doctor.

If lean tissue status cannot be maintained by complete hormone replacement therapy alone, we suggest that an aggressive anabolic steroid program like the ones outlined below be added.

Low-Dose Steroid Cycle for Women

After hormone replacement therapy is determined, the oral anabolic steroid oxandrolone can be used at 2.5 mg to 5 mg two times per day for 12 weeks or until the target body weight is achieved. A small subset of women could experience some virilizing (oily skin, acne, facial hair growth, deeper voice, and itching clitoris followed by clitoral growth) from this normally very safe and gentle steroid. If this happens, reduce the dosage immediately or stop.

Stanozolol in doses of 2 mg to 4 mg two times per day can also be used, but it presents somewhat more potential for virilizing effects.

Higher-Dose Cycles for Women

Higher-dose cycles should be considered for women who need quick increases in lean body mass. Steroid options include oxandrolone,

stanozolol, and nandrolone. We suggest oxandrolone at 20 mg per day for twelve weeks. Or stanozolol can be used at 12 mg per day. If you have a very urgent need to gain lean body mass nandrolone decanoate can be added at 25 to 50 mg per week. Nandrolone does present significantly more potential for virilizing, so monitoring for androgenic side effects is essential if it is used.

Serostim Human Growth Hormone

In the 1980's human growth hormone was the first anabolic drug to be embraced by AIDS activists to address wasting, the number two cause of death in AIDS. At that time media hype and a hysterical anti-drug political climate created an exaggerated image of anabolic steroids as dangerous immunosuppressive drugs that had no legitimate medical uses. For this reason the medical community and some leading AIDS activists rejected any consideration of the use of anabolic steroids and instead attached their hope to GH, which we assert, was a mistake. It is interesting to note that the FDA panel that was to decide whether to approve GH deadlocked because of a lack of convincing data of its effectiveness and only approved it after AIDS activists showed their extreme support. Another interesting point is that it appears that biotech company Genentec decided not to seek approval for their GH product because they did not feel that it would be effective for this use. With all this considered, GH has produced life-saving effects for a few HIV(+) people who were near death and it does have a place in treatment of body composition problems in HIV therapy. While GH does not appear to have a direct effect on muscle tissue growth, it may be that it improves the health of some organ tissues that affect muscle growth, and so some people with severe wasting may experience a small amount of muscle growth, rehydration and improved organ function with GH therapy. However, much of the time it is marketed inappropriately as a muscle builder, where anabolic steroids are far more effective. As will be discussed later, GH's primary value is in its effect on fat cell metabolism.

Comparison of Anabolic Steroids and Growth Hormone

What the following table graphically illustrates is the tremendous disparity between the different anabolic compounds for lean body mass gained versus price. While nandrolone decanoate yielded as much as 11.88 pounds of lean body mass over 15 weeks at a cost of $90 per month, a 6 mg (18 IU) daily dose of Serostim GH, which cost over 100 times more than nandrolone, yielded only a little over half as much lean body mass over 12 weeks. Low doses of other steroids produced equal or better results than Serostim, for much less cost. Even Oxandrin, which is highly overpriced at $900 per month for 20 mg per day outperformed Serostim. Additionally, it is likely that the LBM gained from the steroids consisted of considerably more muscle tissue than what was gained with Serostim. A majority of weight gain from Serostim is generally water. (See the discussion below that is titled *Growth Hormone Gains: Little Muscle, Lots of Water*.)

Choices: Serostim, Oxandrin, Anadrol, or Winstrol

For cost versus weight gain, testosterone and nandrolone are the best anabolic agents without a doubt. Just as it is clear that GH is out of the running in a contest for effect on lean body mass gains, Oxandrin doesn't score much better. Although the men in the Poles study did gain 6.9 pounds of body cell mass on 20 mg of Oxandin per day over 8 weeks, a chart review of wasting HIV(+) males by Dr. Patricia Salvato showed a weight gain of under 2 pounds with 20 mg per day over 12 weeks.[106] Our real world experience is that many male patients need 30 to 50 mg per day of Oxandrin to gain significant LBM if it is used alone. A 30 to 50 mg daily dose of Oxandrin costs *$1.50 per milligram* or $1350 to $2250 per month in the U.S. Oxandrolone (or any steroid) will produce much better results if combined with testosterone, and a very tightly controlled 8 week study by Strawford that included comprehensive weight training showed that 10 mg twice per day with 100 mg of testosterone increased lean body mass by 15.18 pounds compared to 8.36 pounds for testosterone alone with weights. We note that 100 mg of testosterone alone producing 8.36 pounds of weight gain is exceptional – this has never been seen before in any study of testosterone like this. We know these researchers to be the very best at creating tightly controlled studies, and the results of this study were exceptional most probably because the authors did an exceptional job creating it and executing it, so comparison of the results of this study to others is difficult. Our real world experience is that oxandrolone is the weakest of the available anabolic steroids, and this opinion is supported by an overview of the results of all the other studies of oxandrolone in HIV.

The only HIV study of the most potent oral anabolic steroid Anadrol does not give good representation of its cost versus benefit. The 1996 Hengge study of 30 patients over 30 weeks showed that 150 mg per day of Anadrol produced an average of 18 pounds of weight gain. It should also be noted that the subjects in the Hengge study continued to gain weight, even during periods of illness. Anadrol, at this dose would cost $1080 per month in the U.S. However, these numbers are somewhat confusing. *At 24 cents per milligram Anadrol is the most cost-effective oral anabolic steroid,* and a 150 mg daily dose is not necessary for the majority of HIV(+) males. It is likely that at 25 mg/day ($180 per month) or 50 mg/day ($360 per month) Anadrol can increase lean body mass equal to or better than equal doses of Oxandrin, and easily exceed any anabolic effect of GH, but at a much lower cost than either of these compounds. Based on credible anecdotes over many years it is likely that even 10 to 20 mg of Anadrol per day will produce 5 to 10 pounds of lean body mass over 12 weeks. If weight training were included, the lean body mass gain could be even more impressive. Hopefully, UNIMED will study this soon.

Comparison of U.S. Anabolic Agents: Cost Versus Weight Gain

Anabolic Agent Reference Number	Author Year	Study Length In Weeks	Number of Subjects	Exer-cise	Dose (mg)	Average Weight Gain in Pounds	Cost per Month
Testosterone 143	Strawford 1999	8	24	Yes	100 mg/week	8.36 – LBM	$12
Nandrolone 58	1996	16	17	Yes	100 mg every 2 weeks	6.6 — Wt	$30
Nandrolone 98	Bucher 1996	12	73	No	100mg/week	5 — BCM	$60
Testosterone Enanthate 72	Bhasin 1996 (non-HIV)	10	43	Yes	600 mg/week	13.42 — LBM	$48
Nandrolone & Testosterone 106	Salvato 1997	12	20	No	Escalating-De-escalating 100-700 mg/week	13 — Wt	$165 Average
Nandrolone 99	Strawford 1997 2 phases	1st phase 3 wks 2nd phase 12 wks	18	No	1rst — 195 mg per week (3 wks), then 2nd — 200 mg every 2 weeks	1st - 5.28 2nd - 6.6 Total 11.88 LBM	$90 Average
Winstrol 15	Berger 1993	10	1	No	6 mg/day	10 - Wt	$72
Winstrol 15	Berger 1993	4	1	No	6 mg/day	3.5 — Wt	$72
Oxandrin 96	Poles 1997	8	21	No	20 mg/day	6.9 — BCM	$900
Oxandrin & Testosterone 143	Strawford 1999	8	24	Yes	20mg/day 100 mg/ week	15.18 – LBM	$920
Anadrol 100	Hengge 1996	30	30	No	150 mg/day	18 - Wt	$1080
Serostim GH 70	Schambelan 1996	12	178	No	6 mg/day	6.6 — LBM	$6000

Some studies report only total weight (Wt), not lean body mass (LBM) or body cell mass (BCM). Given this, we present the limited available data. Note: BCM is the metabolically active protein tissue and water that are contained in muscle and organs like the heart, liver, and kidneys. LBM includes BCM, extracellular water and bone. Total weight includes LBM and fat.

While Anadrol has a reputation for being a powerful steroid with a significant potential for side effects and liver toxicity, its historic use has been in ultra-high daily doses of 100 mg or more for long periods of time as a treatment for anemia. It is likely that any oral anabolic steroid used long term at ultra high doses will produce side effects and toxicity that won't be seen short term at lower doses. Used in a low dose of 25 mg per day in 12 week cycles the potential for side effects is reduced considerably, while low doses will still promote significant weight gain. The 50 mg Anadrol tablets are scored in half, so consider splitting the tablet into doses of 1/4 tablet and take 1/4 tablet two or three times per day if you choose to try a low dose. (Remember, for best effect, oral steroids should be taken in divided doses several times per day, as blood levels decline after only a few hours.) It is likely that even 1/2 tablet per day would produce some muscle gain.

The other oral steroid Winstrol should also be considered because it produces good increases in lean body mass with little potential for side effects at a relatively low cost of *40 cents per milligram*.[15] Berger's study of 6 mg of Winstrol per day showed good weight gain,[15] which suggests that it may produce more anabolic activity than a comparable dose of Oxandrin, as a similar Berger HIV study did not show any weight gain at 5 mg of Oxandrin per day.[117] Winstrol also exerts its greatest effect when combined with testosterone. It also has not exhibited liver toxicity in the few HIV(+) men we know who have used it at standard doses. Unfortunately, Winthrop, the manufacturer of Winstrol in the U.S., has taken no interest in marketing it to the HIV community or supporting studies. For this reason, we rarely hear of doctors prescribing it. We urge Winthrop to perform studies to assess the effectiveness of Winstrol for HIV.

The Politics of Serostim Growth Hormone

While appropriately prescribed human growth hormone can be another valuable tool in HIV-ther-apy for the war against wasting and especially lipodystrophy, we have considerable philosophical problems with the financial politics related to GH, and are quite critical of its exorbitant price and the deceptive way that it is marketed to the HIV community. Serostim, the GH product that has been approved for AIDS wasting therapy, costs over $6000 per month for a full 6 mg daily dose. This is about 40 times as expensive as the PoWeR cycle that employs high doses of testosterone and nandrolone. But is GH as effective for lean body mass gains for HIV(+) people? The study comparison table above indicates that it is not. We also underline that Serono's compassionate use program for people who do not have insurance is anything but compassionate. While patient access programs from BTG and Unimed are easy to work with, Serono's program is one of the biggest hoop-jumping contests in the HIV world.

Serostim Growth Hormone Has No Preservative

Even if the high cost of Serostim for the relatively small increase in lean body mass was not important, another problem with Serostim is. Serono omits including a bacteriostatic agent in the sterile water that Serostim is reconstituted with, so it must be used within 24 hours after mixing or thrown away because bacteria might grow in the solution. This makes Serostim much more profitable for Serono, while it effectively takes away your option of reducing common side effects by rationing out part of the vial every day to get a lower side effect-free daily dose.

If Serono did include a preservative like benzyl alcohol or metacresol in the mixing water, then you could use whatever dose was found to be appropriate, and store the unused GH in the refrigerator for up to two weeks. Currently, HIV(+) individuals who cannot tolerate the severe side effects that the full 4, 5, or 6 mg doses can cause may end up throwing away any GH that they cannot use. More drug is wasted and thus more drug is sold.

Serono clearly knows about this issue, as their GH product called Saizen, which is sold in Mexico and Italy and prescribed to children in the U.S., *does* have benzyl alcohol in its mixing water. We had a discussion about this with Serono's director of research almost two years ago and were told that it was too difficult to access an effective preservative. To this day Serono representatives are evasive about the lack of a preservative.

Extending Serostim's Lifespan

One way to correct Serostim's lack of a preservative is to get your doctor to give you a prescription for bacteriostatic water that includes benzyl alcohol (made by Abbott Labs and other companies). An insider at Serono admitted that mixing Serostim with bacteriostatic water would allow it to be used for up to two weeks after mixing. After all Serostim is essentially the same product as their other GH called Saizen, except that Saizen comes with bacteriostatic water that contains benzyl alcohol. Using bacteriostatic water allows you to find your own side effect-free individual daily dose without waste.

Eliminating Side Effects

If GH is given as a replacement hormone to HIV-negative people who are GH deficient or are experiencing an age-related decrease in GH production, the typical daily dose is around .5 mg (1.5 IU) per day. Bodybuilders know about safe, side effect-free doses and typically limit their use of GH to under 1.4 mg (about 4 IU) per day.

Serostim is currently packaged in doses of 4, 5, or 6 mg vials, and a study of the medical literature show that these doses are overdoses for many people. Doses that are this high can cause significant side effects including arthralgia (joint pains), carpal tunnel syndrome, edema (water retention), elevated blood sugar, elevated pancreatic enzymes, gynecomastia, body hair growth, and high blood pressure.

Serono's dosing recommendations are lacking in that they instruct patients to use one full vial per day. If this causes side effects the doctor often tells the person to use the full vial every other day, or use only part of the vial every other day, and throw the rest away. These instructions are inadequate. Doctors who work with GH for anti-aging purposes tell us that GH has very little potential for side effects if it is administered in smaller doses more often, with the best effect being seen with twice-a-day administration. Without the peak blood levels that high doses every other day create, there will be fewer side effects. In general, with any drug, smaller doses given more often work better with fewer side effects than large doses given less often. Our recommendation for best effect is to administer GH first thing in the morning and once before bed. If this is too much trouble, administer it before bedtime.

Growth Hormone and Joint Inflammation

Significant research shows that high dose GH may cause joint pains because it can promote excess super oxide secretion by neutrophils, which causes inflammation.[126][127] This effect has a known association with inflammatory joint problems, such as rheumatoid arthritis,[128] so high dose GH appears to be inducing a state like rheumatoid arthritis.

Richard — A Seemingly Dramatic Response to GH

We have seen a few HIV(+) individuals who have a seemingly tremendous anabolic response to the use of high dose GH, and much more so than they do to anabolic steroids. This can be deceptive.

For instance, one of our close friends named Richard, who is 55 years old and has been extremely progressed in AIDS (several times near death), is an example of a person who appears to have a significant resistance to the effects of anabolic steroids, as steroids have not helped him gain as much lean body mass as some people do. In an attempt to help him gain weight, his doctor put him on Serostim GH, and two weeks after he had started Serostim we were surprised to find that he had gained 18 pounds. (We even thought that we might have to re-assess our somewhat critical position on GH.)

However, a few days into his third week he began to be overwhelmed by the problems he was having with side effects. It seems that because of his hopes that GH would be the magic bullet that it is advertised as, he had down-played the fact that he had been experiencing extreme swelling and pain in his hands and other joints, numbness in his hands and arms when he slept, difficulty breathing when he climbed stairs, and he was unable to sleep on his back because he felt like he was suffocating.

On examination, his doctor found that most of the weight he had gained was water, and determined that he was suffering from severe pulmonary edema (water in the lung tissues), so she immediately admitted him to the hospital. After several critical medical procedures while he was in the hospital — he was almost given open-heart surgery — he recovered to live another day. His doctor said that it is unlikely that she would prescribe Serostim again. We assert that this kind of situation can result from the use of the currently recommended 4, 5, and 6 mg doses that for most people are over-doses of GH, and the fact that there is no preservative in Serostim's formulation, which deters people from lowering their dose to reduce the side effects.

Growth Hormone Gains: Little Muscle, Lots of Water

When all things are considered, it appears that Serono recommends what amounts to an overdose of GH because an ultra-high overdose is necessary to come close to producing lean body mass (LBM) gains that seem to be almost equal to the anabolic effects of low doses of anabolic steroids. Using GH to grow muscle is an incorrect use; the increase in LBM may very well consist primarily of water, with some connective tissue, a little organ tissue, and only a little, if any, muscle tissue.

Indeed, one carefully designed study of high-dose GH with HIV-negative young men used sophisticated techniques to closely examine the composition of the lean tissue gained and concluded that it consisted of lean tissue other than muscle.[111] This could mean water, connective tissue, and organ tissue. At least five other studies with other populations have also shown an increase in LBM, but a lack of muscle growth.[135-139] It should be noted that Dr. Kathleen Mulligan stated that GH-induced lean body mass gains for HIV patients were "comparable" to the healthy HIV(-) controls in her study,[28] so comparisons with studies of HIV(-) subjects may very well be valid.

Indeed, the first HIV study that looked at Serostim using magnetic resonance imaging (MRI), a sophisticated technology that actually looks at what is happening to the body's tissues, indicated that growth hormone may have little or no affect on muscle. At the Third International Conference on Nutrition and HIV Infection at Cannes, France, in April, 1999, Dr. Donald Kotler reported the results of an interim analysis of a 6-month open-label trial of Serostim growth hormone that showed that 6 mg per day did not promote a significant change in muscle tissue during the first 12 weeks in the 8 subjects for whom repeat MRI data were available. It appears that if Serostim does actually increase muscle tissue, it does so erratically and only for a very few HIV(+) people, not for the majority.

Human Growth Hormone and Gynecomastia

Gynecomastia is the growth of breast tissue in men. It is sometimes seen in males who use high doses of anabolic steroids that aromatize into estrogen, as estrogen stimulates breast tissue growth. Gynecomastia appears to be a very rare phenomenon in HIV(+) men, at least partially because impaired insulin-like growth factor-1 (IGF-1) production and GH deficiency are common in HIV,[144 145] and IGF-1 is a necessary cofactor with estrogen for breast tissue growth in gynecomastia.[146] [147] GH stimulates production of IGF-1 by the liver, and our observation is that HIV(+) males who use growth hormone appear to have a much higher incidence of gynecomastia than those who don't. Indeed, older studies with young HIV(-) boys and senior men who receive growth hormone therapy have documented incidence of gynecomastia.[148] [149] GH can also stimulate breast tissue growth by binding to prolactin receptors.[150]

Measurements: Finding the Right GH Dosage

Analysis of the available data causes us to assert that GH should be considered for replacement purposes based on blood tests, rather than as a muscle growth stimulant, and prescribed accordingly. However no studies have been done to ascertain what blood levels are appropriate for HIV(+) males and females. Until this is done, our suggestion is that the physician consider testing IGF-1, which is a more consistent measurement than plasma GH, and try to arrive at an IGF-1 measurement of approximately 350 ng/mL, which is the target reading for optimal GH replacement for anti-aging purposes. Because hormonal resistance is common in HIV, it is possible that some HIV(+) people will require higher blood levels to experience the potential improvements in fat metabolism and quality of life. To date we have seen doses of between 0.5 mg and 3 mg per day produce optimal effects for HIV(+) men, so we suggest starting at 0.5 mg per day, and retesting to work toward determining an appropriate dose. Also listen to your patient's subjective reports of their status to determine what is optimal, and be willing to experiment until you find what is appropriate.

Growth Hormone's Benefits

While the available data suggests that GH is not anabolic to muscle tissue like anabolic steroids, and it is clear that GH's price and Serono's lack of a preservative do not serve the HIV(+) population, GH does have unique bene-fits. If GH has more effect on increasing the growth of lean tissue other than muscle, as the studies suggest, does it promote the regeneration of organ tissue like the thymus, kidneys, and liver? This is an area that needs to be researched. Wasting in HIV is not limited to muscle tissue, and regeneration of critical organs in the body may be an important reason for GH replacement therapy in HIV. As was said, it may be that the rare anecdotal reports of a small amount of increased muscle growth in severely wasted HIV(+) individuals are the result of improved function of organs that indirectly affect muscle growth.

And while anabolic steroids can reduce the net ratio of fat to muscle that is gained[99] and can have some effect on increasing the loss of fat, GH's most important effect may be its role in fat cell metabolism;[110] it increases lipid oxidation (fat burning),[77] which gives it a role in possible therapies to reduce some of the symptoms of the body-fat redistribution called lipodystrophy. Dr. Gabe Torres has recently documented that GH can reduce bodyfat redistribution and this is an area that we feel should be investigated thoroughly.

However, we caution that GH may increase the loss of subcutaneous fat on the arms, legs, and face, which are also part of the syndrome.

GH's role is also interesting when we consider that a phenomena of early AIDS wasting is the loss of muscle, while fat is gained, described as *de novo lipogenesis* by Dr. Marc Hellerstein.[73] This kind of catabolism of muscle and anabolism of fat is somewhat unique to AIDS, and it may be in part caused by a resistance to GH[78] and reduced production of IGF-1.[29] So GH appears to have a unique role in a problem that is somewhat specific to AIDS.

We also have anecdotal reports that GH use sometimes stops chronic diarrhea. GH is known to increase tissue regeneration in the intestine[133] and improve intestinal water and ion absorption,[134] so this is possible.

GH Combined with Anabolic Steroids

GH may have valuable adjunctive benefits when used to address GH deficiency when it is combined with testosterone replacement therapy. Appropriately-dosed GH replacement may also enhance the effectiveness of any of the PoWeR anabolic steroid cycles, just as nutritional supplementation that addresses nutrient deficiencies does. We invite the research community to consider studying combination therapy that employs GH replacement and anabolic steroids.

Hyperplasia

When GH is added to a regimen of anabolic steroids and weight training it seems that what muscle is gained is more permanent than when anabolic steroids are used alone. This may be because GH's effect of increasing IGF-1 can increase the number of nuclei in muscle cells by causing satellite cells to fuse to adjacent muscle cells or differentiate into muscle cells.[113] This might result in hyperplasia, an increase in the number of muscle cells and hypertrophy, an increase in cell size. Observation of bodybuilders suggests that this effect may be potentiated by proper exercise stimulus, and optimal levels of androgens. (Note: GH used by itself does not appear to produce lasting lean tissue gains after administration is stopped.[112] This would be true if most of the weight that was gained was water.)

Doctor to Doctor

Physicians might be interested in hearing the experience of another physician who is familiar with the use of anabolic steroids as detailed in this chapter. For this, you might call any of several clinicians who are familiar with our approach. These include Houston's Patricia Salvato, MD, (713) 960-7900; Adan Rios, MD, (713) 961-7100; and Shannon Schrader, MD, (713) 520-5537. These doctors report that many patients using the PoWeR cycle have gained 20 to 40 pounds with increased energy and greatly improved quality-of-life in a matter of two to four months without significant side effects.

They also report some improvements in some of the symptoms of lipodystrophy using specific elements of our program including reduced visceral fat and improvements in blood lipids.

Many other physicians in Houston, Los Angeles, Miami, and San Francisco, and other cities are applying anabolic steroid therapy successfully for therapeutically beneficial changes in body composition for their patients with no significant side effects. PoWeR is committed to supplying physicians and patients who are not familiar with anabolic steroids, information about optimal regimens to maximize lean body mass, enhance quality-of-life and immune response, and minimize potential side effects. The time has come for effective, practical, and economical ways to improve body composition and reverse wasting syndrome.

Orthomolecular Nutrition

by Michael Mooney

This section of the book will tell you about nutrition to help improve metabolism so that you can improve your immune response. It also helps you prime your metabolism to respond well to exercise and anabolic hormone therapy so that you can optimally increase or maintain your lean body mass and reduce lipodystrophy or prevent it. New data being collected by several clinicians, including Dr. Jon Kaiser, the author of *Healing HIV*, indicate that optimal orthomolecular nutrition can also improve metabolism in such a way that lower doses of standard AIDS medications will produce better reductions in viral load and improved T cell counts because your body is more responsive and your immune system is more able to participate in your defense. Lower doses can mean less toxic effects over time, and more potential to maintain sensitivity to the drugs without developing resistance to the effects of the drugs. Dr. Kaiser has a number of patients who are doing so well using this kind of approach that they are achieving good health using relatively low doses of simple combinations of some of the older antiviral AIDS medications so that they haven't even had to begin using the most powerful AIDS medications, the protease inhibitors. Building your health with natural tools is a perfect complement to optimize the effects of progressive HIV medicine.

To give this chapter an anchorage I am going to first refer to my father Patrick's SAINTS study, an acronym for Super Nutrition AIDS Information and Nutritional Study that took place in 1993. The study was devised to see if orthomolecular nutrition could benefit people with AIDS. What Patrick did was to provide an orthomolecular diet (I will explain the word orthomolecular in a minute) and supplementation to 25 people for two months while he kept track of various measurements and the participants' subjective feelings of their quality-of-life. This study used some of same dietary supplements I recommend but only lasted a short two months. If you are diligent in using the information in this section to address your own nutritional needs over the long term you could experience even greater success. The dietary suggestions in this section work well as the basis for the best bodybuilding and the best immune health diet, and provides more tools that may help reduce lipodystrophy.

In the SAINTS system, people learned about their own food allergies and how to avoid and reduce the immune burden that food allergies can cause. The single biggest burden on the immune system that everyone is exposed to on a day-to-day basis is thought to be the allergens in the foods we eat. While all healthy foods contain nutrients, they also all generally contain a little bit of what can be considered to be poisons called allergens. The people in the SAINTS study were taught how to select and cook a clean, allergy-free whole natural foods diet individually tailored for each person. They also learned about the most effective nutritional supplementation to help enhance metabolism and improve natural immune response, and I will cover later in this chapter.

What is Orthomolecular?

The word orthomolecular was coined by a two-time Nobel Prize winner, the late Linus Pauling, in the 1960s when he was exploring the beginnings of nutritional medicine with several other science pioneers. "Ortho" means right or correct, or in this case, natural to the human body, and molecular means "of molecules". In this specific case, it means natural or right molecules for the biochemical needs of the human body because the body has been working with these natural ortho-molecules for millions of years. These molecules are simply the same health-giving nutrients we get from food.

Let me put this in perspective by telling you that when my father and I started seriously investigating progressive nutrition in the 1970s, there were only about 300 doctors in the U.S. who practiced some kind of nutritional medicine, and only a handful of scientists like Dr. Pauling who were involved with it. Today there are thousands of doctors in the United States, including doctors who work with HIV(+) people, who use some of these nutritional techniques in their practice.

Higher Nutrient Doses Work Better — The Threshold Effect

What these pioneer doctors were doing was creating a foundation for health by using a diet of whole natural foods at the same time that they supplied these ortho-molecules, like vitamins, to help correct and strengthen human metabolism by giving the body specific, usually higher than RDA (recommended daily allowance) level amounts of these ortho-molecules. This was to make sure that the body did not suffer from any nutrient deficien-

cies so that it could operate at its best. In some cases they found that giving some people extremely high amounts of these ortho-molecules improved certain disease states. I offer to you the hypothesis that there is a threshold effect for nutrients and that some of the nutrients do not produce as much of an effect in lower doses as they do when they are taken in higher doses. For instance, recently it was shown that 1,000 mcg of folic acid significantly reduced colitis and the incidence of precancerous colon cells while 400 mcg was significantly less effective.[1] 1,000 mcg is an unnatural super-physiologic amount, many times as much folic acid as you would find in any single natural food. However, when given in this orthomolecular amount, folic acid helps reduce the potential for several medical problems. Folic acid supplementation becomes even more interesting when we realize that folic acid found in food is about half as well absorbed as folic acid in dietary supplements.

These orthomolecular doctors also attempted to reduce wear and tear on the body by removing specific foods that people were allergic to from their diets. At the same time that orthomolecular nutrition delivers helpful natural molecules and whole foods, it eliminates or reduces problematic molecules, including artificial compounds, toxins, and the allergens that I am going to talk about, to reduce the metabolic burden that any of them might create. What these scientists found was that they could do some amazing things to improve people's health with this approach.

Conventional western or allopathic medicine tends to use toxic drugs to kill microbes; drugs to kill bugs. And while this approach provides benefits in many specific situations, orthomolecular doctors were using ortho-molecules and getting better results for some medical problems than if they would have used drugs. What they found was that if they strengthened metabolism by using these ortho-molecules, much of the time the body would become strong enough that it would conquer the bugs and get rid of them by itself. This is a healthier, non-toxic, no side effect way of getting healthier. This is because these natural ortho-molecules support healthy immune function and the entire metabolism while not causing the side effects that a majority of drugs do. So orthomolecular nutrition gave birth to orthomolecular medicine, which is nutritionally-based medicine. Orthomolecular is back to nature, but optimally so, using a scientifically developed understanding of natural biochemistry.

Orthomolecular medicine is a scientific approach to improving metabolism by using optimum nutrition to balance and strengthen it. This holistic approach involves simple components in a logical system.

> *I caution that while there are a minority of HIV(+) people who get so healthy using ortho-molecular nutrition that they do not even have to use drugs, most of the time standard AIDS medicines are absolutely necessary.* For the majority of people with critical illnesses an integrated approach, where optimal natural nutrition and progressive medical approaches work together will produce the best effect.

Whole Food

For your best immune health, the first consideration about food is to try to stay whole and natural. This means to try to avoid any food that is artificial, not in its natural form, but don't drive yourself crazy by being too strict about this too quickly. Ease into it if you have to. The important thing is to make it easy for yourself and take it one step at a time. So try to clean your diet up gradually and consistently and use more natural whole foods when you make your selections at the market or restaurant. You will do a lot to improve your health if you only do one thing: gradually add more whole natural foods to your diet, as you remove processed or artificially-created foods. But one step at a time, always. There is an old Chinese proverb that basically means revolutions do not produce lasting change, but gradual adjustments do. (Source: *I Ching: Ting, The Cauldron*)

Fresh Produce

You should take dietary supplements too, but there are as yet undiscovered life-giving nutrients and therapeutic ingredients in vegetables and fruits that show themselves as the variety of colors we see in fresh produce. The produce section of the market is basically a fresh vitamin department and a medicine chest. And while most foods give you simple nourishment, some like garlic, onions, and ginger have genuine therapeutic effects. Eating the widest variety of fresh produce on a daily basis assures you of getting all the ingredients that nature provides that can help keep your body strong enough to handle bacteria and viruses so that you stay healthy.

Besides the fact that organic produce generally has more nutrient content than non-organic, one reason I recommend organic produce is because the chemicals like pesticides that can be found on non-organic produce can negatively impact the immune system. Even if you eat organic produce, always wash your produce well, not only to get the pesticides and chemicals off of the non organic produce, but to get the microorganisms off of any produce. There are lots of tiny bugs living on the surface of fresh produce, and some of them are pretty nasty to a compromised immune system, so wash produce well. To be extra sure the bugs are gone, you should wash your produce with one of the mild organic dish-washing liquids that are sold in natural foods stores. There are also produce cleansers like Healthy Harvest Fruit and Vegetable Rinse that help remove contaminants, like waxes, and pesticides, while destroying common bacteria and fungus. This is especially important if you have low T cells (below 50). Whether the produce you eat is organic or not though, be sure to eat fresh vegetables and fruits on a daily basis as much as possible.

Diet and Allergens

Is "Natural" Always Good?

In natural foods we find that there are components that are good for us and some things that are not so good. The good things are nutrients and some of the primary bad things are the allergens that are found in many of the foods we eat. Just as nature has toadstools and tigers that can kill us, so it is with natural food allergens. Reducing exposure to food allergens reduces a powerful burden on the immune system that sometimes has a profound effect. Two common benefits are a significant reduction in diarrhea, and a tremendous increase in energy. Allergens come in a variety of molecular forms, but what they have in common is that they produce a reaction that stresses your immune system, which responds to it and spends energy dealing with it. So food allergens are something to be avoided. How do we avoid them? There are several methods to detect these allergens, and several ways to handle them once we do.

Four-Day Rotating Diet

One of the easiest ways to handle allergens is to just rotate your foods so that you do not eat from the same food family more than once every four days. With this method, unless you are severely allergic to some food, you will not even have to sleuth out which foods you are actually allergic to. This is called a four-day rotating diet and there are a number of books that tell you all about it. The common allergens that you would rotate or avoid include some of the world's most popular foods: wheat, corn, milk/dairy, bananas, yeast (beer), peanuts, chocolate, tomatoes, citrus, soy, and coffee. Sounds like many people's shopping list, doesn't it? The important thing to remember is to rotate your foods so you do not eat the same ones regularly. You benefit in many ways because you end up getting a variety of different kinds of food and a wider variety of nutrients.

How Do You Know What You Are Allergic To?

Do you say to yourself that a symptom like diarrhea is *"just because I have AIDS?"* Sometimes someone who is HIV(+) will have diarrhea of unknown origin and the standard medical tests will not be able to tell what is causing it, so it is dubbed *"HIV enteropathy."* This is a classic time to look for hidden food allergies.

Food allergies can cause this kind of upset in the gastrointestinal system very easily, without cryptosporidium, or amoebas, or any other pathogen. How do we find out what we are allergic to? The best thing to do is look for cause and effect. This is where the elimination diet can help you find out what you are allergic to.

Food Allergy Rule of Thumb #1: Look For Cause and Effect

1. If I drink milk do I — get diarrhea later that day or get mucus right away?
2. If I eat wheat do I — feel depressed two hours later, or get headaches?
3. If eat tomatoes do I — get skin rashes the next day?

These are some of the kind of reactions to food allergens that are common.

Solutions:

These are the solutions commonly used to detect food allergies so that you can change your diet accordingly. The easiest is item one and the best is item three.

1. Just avoid the most common allergens listed above and rotate your foods. See also the Food Allergen Chart on the next page.
2. Self-test yourself: Read any book on the subject and follow instructions to self-test for allergens. Books include *Dr. Mandell's 5-Day Allergy Relief System*, *Do It Yourself Allergy Analysis* by Ludeman, and *Are You Allergic* by Crook. This is a partial list; there are a lot more books at natural food stores. Then keep a personal food allergy journal and look for cause and effect. Eliminating foods that are suspected of causing allergies one by one can tell you a lot about what causes your problems. Also, for a look at an interesting theory about why different people are allergic to different foods read the book *Eat Right For Your Blood Type*, by Dr. Peter D'Adamo.
3. Get professional allergy screening, which is a clinical test procedure that can give you an assessment of your food allergies

FOOD ALLERGEN CHART

This list presents the most allergenic foods by food group. Individuals will vary in exactly how they react to different foods, as allergenicity depends on many factors, including frequency of exposure to the food, and genetics. If your ancestors evolved eating a given food, there is usually less potential that you are allergic to it. The foods that are most commonly allergenic are listed at the top of the table. Less commonly allergenic ones are at the bottom.

ANIMAL PRODUCTS	VEGETABLES	NUTS/SEEDS	FRUITS	GRAINS
Egg	Tomato Spinach	Peanut Hazelnut (filbert)	Strawberry Fig Mango Raspberry Orange	Wheat Semolina Bulgar Triticale Spelt
Skim milk	Celery (raw) Carrot (raw) Green pea Beans Cabbage (core)	Walnut Pecan Brazil nut Almond	Apple (raw) Apricot (raw) Peach (raw) Date	Corn
Shellfish - Crab - Lobster - Prawn/shrimp - Clam - Oyster	Cauliflower Brussels sprouts Green bean	Cocoa bean Chocolate Coconut	Cantaloupe Raisin Pineapple Apple (cooked)	Oats
Goat cheese	Avocado Cabbage (outer leaves)	Cashew Pistachio Macadamia	Cherry Kiwi Plum/prune Apricot (cooked)	Rye/Barley
Cheese	Onions	Legumes - Soy - Dried peas - Lentils - Dried beans - Navy - Pinto - Garbanzo	Loganberry Boysenberry	Rice
Fin fish - Cod - Sole/whitefish - Tuna - Salmon	Celery (cooked) Green/red Peppers		Banana Grape	Quinoa
Ham Pork	Potato Cucumber Lettuce	Sesame seed Pumpkin seed	Grapefruit Lemon Lime	Buckwheat
Chicken Beef	Asparagus Broccoli Beets		Watermelon Currants	Amaranth
Buttermilk Yogurt	Squash	Carob	Peach (cooked/canned)	Arrowroot
Wild game - Deer - Elk - Moose - Buffalo	Carrot (cooked) Parsnip	Bean sprouts	Cranberry Blackberry Blueberry	Millet
Butter	Turnip Sweet potato Yam		Pear	
Turkey Lamb Rabbit			Rhubarb	

with less effort on your part. If your doctor does not know how to do this, they should be able to refer you to specialists who are geared to do this. Several of the best tests are the Serammune physicians' Elisa/ACT, functional assessment tests like the liver detoxification panel, Great Smokies digestive analysis tests, and the intestinal permeability test. Ask your physician, registered dietitian, or certified nutritionist if they know about these tests.

The Components of Whole Food

Foods are made up of many different components, some are micro or small nutrients, like vitamins, and some are macro or large nutrients. The three macro groups that compose the majority of our diets are carbohydrates, proteins and fats. These three units are the basic materials that fuel our activities and maintain our lean body mass. Selecting the best sources of these three helps to optimize body composition and prevent muscle loss and bodyfat accumulation and dysfunction.

The Best Carbohydrates

Carbohydrates provide our body's main source of quick energy. After carbohydrates are digested and after some processing by the liver, they are released into the blood stream as a sugar called glucose to be delivered to the cells.

Throughout the majority of the last million years of our evolution the human diet consisted of animal carcasses, some seeds, nuts, and fibrous vegetable and fruit carbohydrate sources that are generally nutrient-rich with lots of water, but are not calorie dense. E.g. they typically contain 150 to 450 calories per pound. The majority of these carbohydrate sources are vegetables, leaves, roots, and fruits. Because the vegetable fiber tends to slow down digestion, or a majority of the carbohydrates in these foods are digested relatively slowly, the moderate amount of sugar that is released from these foods doesn't produce profound lasting effects on blood sugar. (Note: fruits have carbohydrates that release relatively quickly, but the net amount of carbohydrates is still not great.)

It was only about 10,000 years ago, which is not very long on the evolutionary scale, that human beings were introduced to high intakes of grains as carbohydrate sources with the advent of agriculture. The problem with high intakes of grains is that grains deliver lots of calories (energy), approximately 1,200 to 1,600 calories per pound. Additionally, some grains deliver their sugar energy relatively quickly, especially if the grain is milled, as are breads and pasta. When a large amount of sugar energy is released into the blood stream it creates a dysfunctional hormonal environment that can ultimately promote several of the diseases that we associate with modern society, including obesity, cardiovascular disease, and diabetes. This hormonal shift also has a profound affect on muscle and fat metabolism, and immune (T cell) function. The key hormone involved in this problem is called insulin, produced by an organ called the pancreas.

Insulin and Insulin Resistance

As was discussed in the chapter on lipodystrophy, insulin's main job in the body is to promote the delivery of sugar energy as glucose to cells. When a small amount of glucose is delivered into the blood stream, a small amount of insulin is produced by the pancreas to accompany it. When there is a large amount of glucose, the pancreas works to produce a large amount of insulin to facilitate its delivery so that cells can take in as much glucose as is possible. Extra glucose that cannot be taken in by the cells circulates in the blood stream, and under normal circumstances most of it is soon converted into triglycerides (fat) so that the unused energy can be stored.

The correct amount of healthy carbohydrate sources will provide enough sugar to give a healthy amount of glucose to the cells, but not too much at once, so that levels of glucose and insulin in the blood stream are not unusually elevated for any long time period. The pancreas works, but it is not overworked trying to keep up with an unusual demand for insulin. However, in modern American society, much of the diet consists not only of large amounts of high calorie carbohydrate sources, such as grains like wheat and corn, but carbohydrates from sweets, which are very concentrated sources of sugar. The net effect that intake of these calorie-dense carbohydrate foods creates is a blood stream that is occasionally flooded with large amounts of glucose, a pancreas that is overworked, and large amounts of insulin and triglycerides circulating in the blood stream. Note that excess insulin causes increased production of cholesterol.

Over time, these occasional glucose, triglyceride and insulin floods can cause a decrease in the sensitivity of the cell's response to insulin, which reduces the cell's ability to take in glucose. This is similar to what would happen if you listened to extremely loud rock music, or worked on jet engines frequently over several years; after a while your hearing, which is normally sensitivity to sound, would suffer, and you would become insensitive to noise. Insensitivity to insulin is called insulin resistance, and it is a serious consideration in HIV because we are now seeing it as one of the core component of bodyfat redistribution syndrome, also known as lipodystrophy, which was addressed earlier.

This is why it is best to select the majority of your carbohydrate intake from slow-releasing carbohydrate sources that do not contain an excessive amount of calories. You will have less potential for insulin resistance, and you will find that you grow muscle more easily when your insulin mechanism is healthy.

Carbohydrate Pecking Order

This is the suggested pecking order of carbohydrate food sources that shows you which carbohydrate sources support your health without increasing insulin resistance. Best are vegetables in their many forms. Raw or steamed vegetables should be included whenever you eat. They are foundation materials and basically cannot be overconsumed. It is almost impossible to get fat eating vegetables, unless they are cooked in oil. Then come fruits; the sweetest ones should be eaten somewhat sparingly if bodyfat is a problem, and the best times to eat them are first thing in the morning or right after a workout when insulin sensitivity is high. Bananas are among the fruits to be moderate with if bodyfat is a problem, because they are among the sweetest, most fattening of fruits. Next are beans and peas. These deliver more calories than vegetables, but the carbohydrates release relatively slowly, much more slowly than grains. Next are whole grains, including oatmeal, barley, and rye, which are calorie dense, but contain carbohydrates that generally release slowly. At the very bottom and the most likely to promote bodyfat problems are carbohydrates from grains, like wheat, and corn. Whole grains are marginally better than processed grains, but when they are milled into flour the difference is not that great. The very worst carbohydrate sources are sweets, like candies.

I suggest that people reduce the use of wheat in general, even whole wheat, and especially if the wheat is in milled form, like flour or bread. When wheat is milled, the carbohydrates it contains digest and convert to sugar very quickly. This can produce a quick rise in blood sugar, even more quickly than white table sugar.[69]

The gluten in wheat and other grains has also been shown to increase the incidence of neuropathy in normal populations.[106]

Try to eat from the first group of slow-release carbohydrate sources a majority of the time, and if you are relatively healthy, with no lipodystrophy, you can cheat once in a while and even have a little milled wheat products or sweets.

My dietitian friends remind me that some HIV(+) people who have weight-loss problems need all the calories they can get, and I agree that this is a sensitive area that requires some delicate balancing, so each person should consider their own situation carefully. But remember, if you have a problem with too much bodyfat or bodyfat redistribution, elevated blood glucose, elevated triglycerides or elevated cholesterol, high-calorie starchy carbohydrates from foods like pasta and bread can be your worst enemy.

Timing Meals for Best Muscle Growth

For bodybuilding purposes there is a time when it is advantageous to allow blood sugar to elevate so that insulin helps the muscle-growing process. This means timing meals that contain carbohydrates, and especially simple carbohydrates, for best modulation of natural insulin production to enhance muscle growth. The simplest and best suggestion is to drink a high-carbohydrate, high-protein low-or non-fat bodybuilding drink immediately after weight-training, as this is the time when a rapid rise in insulin levels will drive the carbohydrates and amino acids into the muscle cells. After the drain of exercise, the body can be basically starved for carbohydrates and amino acids and is primed to transport them into the muscles more efficiently, with less potential for the calories to spill over and be transformed into fat for storage. A rapid rise in insulin to enhance energy delivery at this time is desirable to enhance muscle growth. This after-exercise meal could also be the highest-calorie meal of the day.

Combining Carbohydrates with Protein, Fiber and Fat

If you eat carbohydrates at the same time that you eat protein, fiber or fat, the digestion of the carbohydrates will be slower, which helps to reduce the rise in blood sugar. However, it is better just to reduce the overall intake of starches and sugars, and I note that the combination of starchy carbohydrates or sweets with fats causes us to gain more body fat than any other combination. (Think ice cream or pizza.) Neither fat nor carbohydrates alone will produce as much of a problem as this combination, so keep this in mind if you want to lose body fat.

The Glycemic Index of Various Carbohydrates

Most of the time, try to eat below 69 percent on the scale below. This glycemic index tells us basically how much a carbohydrate raises blood sugar and upsets the insulin balance when eaten by itself. The higher the percentage, the greater the rise in blood sugar. Notice how sweet foods, or foods that release sugar quickly, are at the top. Also note, in real-world situations carbohydrates are usually combined with fiber, protein, and fat. Combinations tend to reduce the effect that carbohydrates can have on blood sugar, and so this table is only a reference point. Foods high on this chart can increase the potential for insulin resistance, diabetes, atherosclerosis, and perhaps lipodystrophy, especially when eaten in quantity. If you do eat them, be sparing.

Sweeteners

Nutrasweet/aspartame — Aspartame is used in most of the top-selling protein powder drink mixes because it replaces sugar as a sweetener

---

Glycemic Index Scale

100% - Glucose
80-90 % - Honey, fruit juices, corn flakes, carrot juice, instant mashed potatoes or rice, raisins, cream of wheat
70-79% - White bread, white rice, whole wheat bread, pasta, bananas
60-69% - Brown rice, green peas, grapes, yams, oranges
50-59% - Apples, pear, oatmeal, cream of rye
40-49% - Milk, lima beans, navy beans, cherries
30-39% - Lentils
10-29% - Low-fat yogurt (unsweetened), soybeans, peanuts, fructose*

---

*While fructose is low on this scale, fructose raises cholesterol, promotes insulin resistance, and stores more readily as fat than other sugars. *Read food ingredient labels and try to reduce the intake of fructose and high-fructose corn syrup.*

so the drink can give you muscle-building protein without giving you fat-making sugar, and still taste sweet. There are two sides to the aspartame story, though.

People with a genetic disease called phenylketonuria get what amounts to toxic reactions from aspartame. Another small percentage of the population appear to have a tendency towards having phenylketonuria. If you are one of these people, you may get headaches, dizziness, or nervous system problems from aspartame. There have also been numerous reports from the general population to the Food and Drug Administration of reactions to aspartame that resemble poisoning of the nervous system, with symptoms like blindness, dizziness and multiple sclerosis-like effects occurring. Whether aspartame is truly toxic or not is controversial, but I personally avoid this totally unnatural molecule.

If you have bodyfat problems try to minimize sweetening with sugar and honey, or natural brown sugar, because *all* sugary sweeteners can upset the insulin balance.

The Food and Drug Administration recently approved a new sugar substitute called sucralose that appears to be non-toxic, but tastes like sugar. It's a chlorinated version of sucrose. The chlorination prevents it from being metabolized, so it does not deliver calories or raise blood sugar. This might just become the most widely used sweetener in the world over the next few years. I do not know if it is really totally safe, though.

Fats and Oils

There are a number of different kinds of fats. There is motor oil, there is butter, and there are essential fatty acids. The most important oil to keep a Honda running right is *not* essential fatty acids (EFAs), but if you want to help your body stay healthy, and your immune system keep operating at its best, you had better consider getting these EFAs on a daily basis. They are called essential because your body can not manufacture them. They are necessary for every

critical function in your metabolism including building muscle and fighting infections. EFAs are one of the reasons I do not advocate a super low-fat diet.

I recommend that you read a couple of books on diet that include more healthy fat than the older diets used to recommend. Probably the most popular book on the subject is *Mastering The Zone*, by Barry Sears, which is available at most book stores; this is Dr. Sears' second book on the so-called "zone" diet. *I have heard several people on protease inhibitors say that the zone diet was the only thing that caused their elevated cholesterol levels to normalize.* Another book that uses the same zone type principles, but is a little easier to follow, is *The Fat-Burning Diet*, by Jay Robb. (Cost: $12.99 plus shipping; to order call 1-800-862-8763.) Do not let the title fool you. The Fat-Burning Diet could be modified a little and be called *the Fat Burning, Muscle Building Diet*. Both *The Fat-Burning Diet* and *Mastering the Zone* will help you build muscle, too, if you get enough calories. Both books support a balanced healthy approach to diet that can help you build muscle and reduce fat. But be careful to eat more calories than they recommend for losing fat if you want to build muscle.

The main point is that since we need EFAs and other fats for health, we should be getting them in our diets from fresh high-quality sources. The diet I am proposing reduces the amount of starchy carbohydrates in the diet, while maintaining a certain amount of healthy fats so that there is a different macronutrient balance than the old high-carbohydrate, high-protein, low-fat diets contained. This means striving to get fatty acids from several fatty acid sources, the least of these are the saturated fats that we find in butter or animal fat. Understand that saturated fats are not the demons we have been led to believe. When we realize that we evolved getting a certain amount of saturated fat from foods in the wild it is only logical that they would have a place in a healthy diet. One recent study showed that dietary saturated fats, and monounsaturated fats were associated with healthy testosterone production in humans, while EFAs had no effect,[5] so it appears that we need a little saturated fat for optimal hormonal health However, most people get far too much saturated fats, which promote insulin resistance and perhaps lipodystrophy, and not enough EFAs, which are needed for the health of the cells and the healthy function of the immune system.

The other important kind of fat that we should consciously include in our daily diet are the mono-unsaturated fats, which we get from foods like olive oil. Recent data has shown that mono-unsaturated fats decrease the risk of certain cancers, and have an anti-inflammatory effect.[33] AIDS is an inflammatory disease, so mono-unsaturated fat intake logically has a place of importance in AIDS, too.

Fats are also a good source of energy needed for muscle growth. They contain nine calories per gram, compared to only four calories per gram for carbohydrates and protein. *It is much more difficult to gain muscle on a low-fat diet.* Low-fat diets are sometimes necessary for HIV(+) people who have compromised digestive systems, but they are not adequate for optimal muscle growth for HIV(+) people who can digest fats.

Fatty Acid Recommendations

I recommend that you consider supplementing your diet with essential fatty acids as per the recommendations I give in the dietary supplement section. EFAs include the omega-3 and omega-6 fatty acids. Most people get an imbalance of these

---

Important Warning!

HIV(+) individuals should be sure that their digestive system is stable and healthy before increasing the amount of dietary fats. Increases in fats for HIV(+) people with compromised digestion can cause serious problems. Diarrhea tends to worsen on a higher fat diet. But keep in mind that medicines like Norvir and Fortovase/Saquinavir need to be taken with higher amounts of fat.

---

two by consuming too little omega-3 fats, which have anti-inflammatory properties, and relatively too much omega-6 fats, which tend to promote inflammation when out of balance. To get more omega-3's, eat more fish, including salmon, tuna, sardines, anchovies, mackerel, rainbow trout, and herring. Omega-6's are contained in common vegetable oils, like sunflower, safflower and corn oils. Try to reduce your intake of these.

Studies show a decrease in tumor necrosis factor and IL-1, a catabolic cytokine associated with wasting, with optimal intake of the omega-3 fatty acids that are contained in fish oils.[6]

Oils and Cooking

Olive oil is one of the best oils to cook with. You can also cook with high-oleic sunflower oil, avocado, canola or any oil that is high in mono-unsaturated fatty acids.

Avoid heating lighter-weight oils like corn and sesame. These oils contain more omega-6 fats, and less mono-unsaturated fats, so they have a higher potential for spoiling and turning to trans fats, which are bad for the immune system. Try to avoid any intake of these lighter oils when they are not absolutely fresh.

Also, choose oils that are minimally processed. Most of the clear oils in the supermarkets are stripped of some of their natural components, because stripping them makes them more suitable for sitting on store shelves for long periods of time without spoiling. *Do not use these stripped oils.* Buy natural food brands like Spectrum Naturals and Hain. And when you do cook, do not overheat the oil so that it smokes. Smoking causes the formation of carcinogens, and destroys the beneficial fatty acids.

You can use a small amount of saturated animal fat like butter to cook, as these fats do not have the potential for converting to trans fatty acids like vegetable oils do. In fact, they are in some ways much safer to cook with than most vegetable oils.

For a guide that details the different types of fats in different oils and which oils can be heated, call Spectrum Naturals at 1-800-995-2705 or 1-707-778-8900, and ask for a copy of their *Kitchen Guide To Oils*.

Avoid Margarine, Hydrogenated Fats or Processed Oils

Do your best to avoid processed fats or oils as they have negative effects on cellular health, overall metabolism, and your immune system. Look out for the words hydrogenated and partially-hydrogenated. These kinds of manipulated fats probably *do* increase the risk of cancer and heart disease. They also weaken healthy cellular immune metabolism, which means that they might increase HIV progression. And lastly, they are also likely to promote lipodystrophy.

Digestion Of Fats

You may need digestive enzymes like lipase to help your digestive system break down fats efficiently. If you have a problem with digestion of fats or digestion in general, you might try taking a supplement that contains lipase (fat-digesting enzymes) or mixed digestive enzymes that include lipase to see if this will help.

Protein Pecking Order

Dairy proteins are at the top of the list of proteins that optimally feed muscle growth. The amino acid balances, insulinogenic potential[25] and overall growth factor content add up to one thing; *milk proteins were created to make mammals grow bigger.* While there is a lot of hoopla related to which dairy protein fractions are best, there is more misunderstanding than reality in this area.

If you are not allergic to dairy protein, or are lactose intolerant, for best muscle growth, I recommend supplementing your regular food protein intake with a dairy protein powder supplement at 50 to 100 grams per day. In general, dairy proteins appear to be somewhat better for gaining muscle than egg or soy protein powders. I say this based on personal experience, but knowing that the real differences may not be that great if there is enough total protein in the diet. In fact, the idea that any one protein is superior is challenged by a small short-term study by Lowery, Ziegenfuss and Appicelli that was reported in issue number 5 of Peak Training Journal (fall 1998). This study showed that when weight-lifting subjects ingested soy, ion-exchange-filtered whey, gel-filtered whey or caseine, there appeared to be a trend towards a very slight advantage for caseine, but it was not clear that the advantage was significant. This study suffered because of its short length, so more investigation needs to be done to get a clearer picture of what differences there really are.

One of the things that will probably produce the most noticeable effect on muscle growth is to make sure you take in a lot of quick-digesting protein immediately after working out, along with the critically important carbohydrates, but little, if any, fat. This is the time when the body is primed for anabolic activity,[50,51] so feed it well.

Whey Protein Myths

For simply gaining muscle, any of the quality brand name bodybuilding dairy protein powders, like Jarrow's American Whey Protein, SportsPharma Just Whey, Champion's Pure Whey, Osmo's Whey, Next Nutrition Designer Protein, and Solgar's Whey To Go are all probably equivalent. I believe that when we are concerned about how much muscle these proteins will help us gain, the differences between the whey products are highly exaggerated. If someone ever did a placebo-controlled blinded study to examine which whey protein enables more muscle gain, I think that there would probably be no significant difference between the various products. Additionally, a hard look at the scientific literature tells us that in spite of the whey hype in the bodybuilding marketplace, whey is probably not the singular best protein for building muscles.

Several of the whey companies say in their advertisements that they have a big advantage over another whey product because they are hydrolyzed, or they are filtered in some high-tech way, or they have more glutamine, etc.

From the lab tests I have seen, some of these claims are simply false. One set of lab tests of three top whey products showed that none of them were actually hydrolyzed, though they all claimed they were hydrolyzed on their labels and in their ads. Additionally, their glutamine contents were highly exaggerated.

I will admit that I too recommended whey for muscle growth previously, and made the mistake of taking whey's superiority for granted based on limited information (not studying this subject thoroughly) and the recommendations of "experts" in the field. The lesson is do not take anything for granted, and every expert makes mistakes, usually in not being thorough enough

Cottage Cheese and Caseine

The truth is, when the totality of scientific data is considered, the old standard dairy protein called caseine looks to be a better muscle-building protein than whey because of two things. Studies show that it is retained in the body better than whey because of physiochemical characteristics specific to caseine,[61] and because caseine has at least 60 percent more L-glutamine than whey. L-glutamine is definitely one of the single most important nutrients if your goal is to grow muscle and prevent its breakdown.

My advice for simplest, best muscle-building protein supplementation, is to eat cottage cheese, a rich source of caseine and glutamine, and/or use protein powders that contain caseinates. It is also likely that the very best protein for muscle growth would contain a natural mix of both casein and a little whey — similar to milk's natural balance.

Medical-Grade Whey Proteins

For therapeutic protein needs, whey proteins can be specially engineered to help improve their potential to benefit immune function and reduce diarrhea. Both of these benefits will help you put on muscle weight and be healthier. There are two medical-grade whey protein powders that are manufactured to cause these kinds

of beneficial effects, Immunocal and Optimune, although the less expensive bodybuilding whey products will produce these effects to some extent, too. What separates Immunocal and Optimune from the less expensive wheys is the fact that they are manufactured to have high amounts of specific protein fractions that purposely address medical needs.

Immunocal

There are more published studies on Immunocal than any other protein product, and the data are strong enough that it deserves consideration by HIV(+) people *who can afford it*. It cost $99 per month but can be found at a discount for about $70, so it is expensive. However, its value is not as a bulk muscle building protein, but as a tool to increase glutathione, an antioxidant your body makes that is critically important for immune function and long-term survival. (Glutathione is discussed in the section on dietary supplements.)

One small, but interesting study, showed that over a three-month period, HIV subjects using Immunocal gained between 4 and 15 pounds without anabolic steroids.[23] Immunocal has also been shown to increase tissue glutathione levels and glutathione content in blood mononuclear cells,[65-67] because it contains high levels of glutamyl-cysteine, a molecule that contains the amino acids glutamine and cysteine. Immunocal appears to raise glutathione much better than the common bodybuilding whey proteins. This is because the manufacturer takes great pains to protect the glutamyl-cysteine from excessive heat or processing that would destroy it. They also provide you with a special plastic blade blender that they say will not denature the glutamyl-cysteine the way a typical fast metal blade blender could. Denaturing compromises the molecular structure of glutamyl-cysteine. Keep in mind that hydrolyzing basically destroys glutamyl-cysteine, so whey proteins that are hydrolyzed have significantly less potential to help raise your glutathione production.

Several highly successful bodybuilding companies, have made claims in their ads about the potential immune-boosting effects of their whey protein products by quoting from publications that specifically studied Immunocal, and not their product. Lab test results I have seen show that several leading whey proteins, including Next Nutrition Designer Whey Protein, are not equal to Immunocal for glutathione production. It is likely that none of the whey proteins produced by sports nutrition companies will increase glutathione production as much as Immunocal *in the same doses*.

However, I am not sure that using a greater amount of a less costly bodybuilding whey protein would not produce an effect that is equal to Immunocal, so it might be less costly but just as effective to use a less expensive whey protein. Data show that some of the bodybuilding proteins increase glutathione production about half as much as the same dose of Immunocal.[67] If Immunocal costs about three to five times as much as a bodybuilding whey product, but only increases glutathione a little over twice as much as the less expensive protein, it might be more cost effective to just use more of the bodybuilding whey product. Maybe, maybe not.

Even so, until recently I was very skeptical of Immunocal's claims of its uniqueness and recommended against it because of its cost and the fact that it is so hard to mix in water. However, a close friend of mine, a very skeptical medical doctor with full-blown AIDS, whose viral load is over 500,00, has had such good results with Immunocal that I have had to re-assess it. While the most advanced AIDS medications have generally failed to help this doctor, he told me that he felt a noticeable difference in the way he felt during the first two weeks of Immunocal use, and gained about five pounds. He said, *"The only two things that I have used for my AIDS that really made a difference that I could feel right away were anabolic steroids and Immunocal."* He also said that after a few weeks of Immunocal use he did not notice as much, but he still feels better than before he used it. I recommend that people

with HIV or AIDS experiment with Immunocal and see if it contributes to your well-being and overall health — if you can afford it.

Optimune

The other medical-grade whey protein is called Optimune. There are no controlled HIV studies with Optimune yet (an ACTG study is in process), but what data there are and anecdotes from our clients suggest that it too may benefit people with HIV. Its value is also not as a bulk bodybuilding protein. While the data I have seen suggest that Optimune produces only about half the increase in glutathione that Immunocal does, lab tests confirm that Optimune contains very high levels of immunoglobulins (IGs), similar to IGs in colostrum, which is found in cow's milk during the first few days after birth. Bovine IGs appear to have a therapeutic benefit for reduction of diarrhea because IGs can contribute to local immune function in the intestine.[91] They are employed in the intestine to help the body fight some of the harmful microorganisms that damage the villi in the mucosal lining of the intestine and cause diarrhea and malabsorption of nutrients.[92] Lab tests show that Optimune has over two times as much of an important IG called IGA and greater amounts of several other IGs than what is contained in Next Nutrition Designer Whey Protein. I also have reports of a reduction in the chronic gas that can be caused by protease inhibitors when Optimune and glutamine are taken together. For chronic gas or diarrhea, people are using one scoop of Optimune with one tablespoon of glutamine powder three times per day. However, people who are allergic to dairy may experience more diarrhea when they use Optimune.

Egg Protein

Next on the list are egg proteins. The important thing to remember is that whole egg is probably somewhat better than egg white for muscle growth and overall health effect, because the yolk is a rich nutrient source, and its protein content complements the protein in the egg white. Together they are a better source of protein.

Meat Protein

While real food like meats often seems to take a back seat to protein powders in the mind of the public because of the mindset created by slick advertising, professional bodybuilders and athletes know the value of real food related to muscle growth. If you do not make real food and meat fundamentals in your diet you will not grow muscle tissue as well. Fish, chicken, turkey and beef are vitally important foods for best muscle growth, not just because of the protein content but because they contain numerous other nutritional components that are important for healthy metabolism. The message is — *eat real food*, and then supplement food with protein powder drinks.

Red meat builds blood, and is a superior source of bodybuilding and blood-building nutrients. These include creatine, carnitine, phenylalanine, conjugated linoleic acid (CLA) and heme (blood) iron, the most absorbable form of iron. That may be why some bodybuilding veterans assert that red meat appears to help improve muscle growth and stamina somewhat better than white meats. And meat, in general, is less likely to cause allergic reactions than eggs or dairy proteins, like caseine and whey. The only caution about red meat is that the high amount of saturated fat some red meat contains could promote lipodystrophy because too much saturated fat promotes insulin resistance. So be moderate about including it in your diet and choose leaner meats if you do.

Important details on meat: cooking kills bacteria in meats. Stewed meat is better for digestion (chicken soup, beef stew). Roasting is OK. Try not to fry, or barbecue with charcoal. Charred foods are associated with increased risk of cancer. Any cooking of meat or vegetable protein that causes the formation of a hard outer skin renders the protein that becomes the skin to be much less digestible because it cross-links the protein. Hair is an example of highly cross-linked protein. Hair is protein, but it is not very digestible.

Try to avoid non organic meat because of the potential of being exposed to the antibiotics in non organic meat, which can be immunosuppressive.[10]

Do not go crazy, but when you do have the choice, choose organic foods, and ask for it where you buy your groceries. Consumer demand changes what is sold in stores. I recommend eating leaner meats, but do not stress out by over-avoiding fat. Remember, fat is not altogether bad, but monounsaturated fats are probably best, and some regular intake of polyunsaturated fats from fish, vegetables, nuts and seeds are necessary for the health of the immune system.

Animal Proteins Versus Vegetable Proteins

Animal proteins generally create more insulinogenesis than vegetable proteins, because of differences in insulinogenic amino acid content.[12 25] In this context insulin can be an important part of the muscle growth mechanism.

Vegetable proteins appear to score lower for building muscle, but should be included in a varied diet for optimal health. The amino acid balances in vegetable proteins do not appear to support muscle growth the way animal sources do,[12] but the new designer soy protein powders, like Supro soy protein, are closer to being equal to animal sources.

Vegetarian Diets

It is very difficult to gain lean muscle weight on a vegetarian diet. In fact, it is almost impossible for most people, especially when they are fighting infections that burn lean body mass. While I know a very few HIV(+) people who can do well adhering to a vegetarian regime, I find that the vast majority cannot do it and keep their lean body mass. Additionally, vegetarian diets increase the potential for anemia because of a lack of blood-building components such as highly absorbable heme iron and vitamin B12. Anemia is already a significant problem for HIV(+) people.

If you do choose a vegetarian diet your best protein sources are beans, and seeds and nuts.

Digestion of all nuts and seed will be improved by soaking them overnight. This helps to reduce the antiproteolytic enzymes they contain that inhibit digestion of the proteins. If you can eat them without digestive problems, many nuts and seeds are ideal foods in several ways because they contain protein, healthy fat, and complex carbohydrates in a very good balance for overall health. They also make a great snack between meals. However, the amino acid balances in these proteins do not appear to be optimal for best growth for humans. Maybe that is why people in cultures who rely heavily on nuts and seeds for their protein are usually shorter and smaller than people in other cultures.[11] Again, vegetarian or vegan diets present a challenge to people with HIV or AIDS who need to gain lean body mass for survival. Unless you are vegetarian for ethical reasons consider eating fish.

Protein and Weight-Training

Anabolic hormone therapy is much more affective when a high-protein (approximately one gram of protein per pound of bodyweight per day), slightly hyper-caloric (calories above maintenance level) diet is maintained consistently. Note: Higher protein intake is known to be necessary for the anabolic effect of anabolic steroids.[15]

Caution: People who are on HIV medications like Crixivan or Previon, which greatly burden the kidneys, should be careful about increasing their protein intake, as this can increase the potential for kidney problems. Ask your doctor if you are taking kidney-toxic medicines, and, if so, only eat a higher protein diet under your doctor's direction. Also those with liver problems should be careful about higher protein intake, and should also do so only under your doctor's supervision. It is wise to increase your protein intake very slowly over a couple of weeks, so that your digestive system adjusts. This will help to reduce gas, bloating and other gut problems. Avoid dehydrating liquids like alcohol and caffeine, and drink lots of water.

How Much Protein

One animal study showed that glutathione production decreased when protein intake fell below 20 percent of normal calories. But 40 percent was no better than 20 percent.[13] I recommend about 25 to 30 percent of the diet as protein for best muscle growth and immune health. This leaves a margin for error for impaired digestion. I generally recommend somewhere around 1 gram of protein per pound of body weight per day while you are trying to gain muscle — if your digestive system, and your liver and kidneys are healthy. I find that less than 3/4 of a gram per pound of body weight often times compromises optimal muscle growth if you are training hard with weights.

This agrees with published data from protein researcher Dr. Peter Lemon that indicates that hard training weightlifters will do better when protein intake is approximately .8 grams per pound of body weight.[14] .8 grams is more than double the current RDA protein intake for sedentary people, which is .36 grams per pound of body weight. I have consistently seen higher protein intake produce better results with bodybuilders and other hard-training athletes over many years. It is also consistent with the dietary protein intake of the U.S. National Weight-lifting team in Colorado Springs, based on the research of the sports scientists that work with the weight-lifting team, the athletes get about 1 1/4 grams of protein per pound of bodyweight.

If you do eat higher protein, drinking 8 to 12 eight ounce glasses of water per day helps flush the kidneys.

Dietary Supplements

When it comes to improving your chances of health and survival, nutrients can be as valuable as drugs in some respects, with a thousand times less potential for toxicity or side effects. As I said, Dr. Jon Kaiser believes that good nutritional support may improve your body's response so that lower doses of drugs work better, which means less overall toxicity. He also asserts that you are less likely to develop resistance to the drugs, so you don't have to switch drugs or drug combinations as often. Nutrients also enhance healthy immune response, and can prime your metabolism for best muscle growth. These are compelling reasons to optimize your nutrient program. How do you do this? Fundamentals first. While there a number of exotic dietary supplements and special foods and herbs that may be very helpful, the most important thing to include in your life are high-potency, complete daily multivitamins and minerals. These should include all the essential vitamins and minerals, along with the common antioxidants, as they all support optimal immune health.

You definitely need a lot more than the RDA, though, as a number of studies over the last several years have shown that supplementing with higher doses of specific nutrients improves the potential for survival in HIV. For instance, studies on micronutrient megadoses in HIV disease conducted by Dr. Mariana Baum of the University of Miami School of Medicine found that nutrient abnormalities of vitamins B2, B6, B12, A, C, E, and zinc were prevalent in HIV-1 infected men *despite dietary nutrient intake at or above the RDA.* She also found that HIV(+) people needed *6 to 25 times* the RDA levels of essential nutrients to get healthy cellular levels of these nutrients, some of which are correlative with a decrease in infections and increase in survival.[17][19]

In her study Dr. Baum found that it took about 6 times the RDA of vitamin B2, 10 times the RDA of vitamin B5, 25 times the RDA of vitamin B12, 10 times the RDA of vitamin A, 6 times the RDA of vitamin C, 6 times the RDA of vitamin E, and 6 times the RDA of zinc to get adequate blood levels of these essential survival nutrients. And, very important, no evidence of toxicity was observed at these doses.

You Can Not Get All Your Nutrients From Food

I have heard conservative dietitians say that HIV(+) people should try to get all their nutrients from food, but Dr. Baum's data shows that this is impossible. If we consider that it takes

about 5 servings of fruits and vegetables just to get the RDA of essential nutrients, then it would take somewhere between 30 and 125 servings of fruits and vegetables per day to get what Dr. Baum's data tells us HIV(+) people need. Fortunately, numerous dietitians who work with HIV(+) people go beyond the outdated conservative approach to nutrition and recommend a progressive approach to supplementing the diet with vitamins.

And while the medical community has done great work in learning to control viral replication and increase T cells during the last few years, they are generally still behind the times when it comes to the importance of nutrient supplementation. At a lecture at the Wasting Therapies and AIDS conference in New York several years ago one well-known doctor told 400 HIV(+) people that *"Unless your T cells are below 500, you don't need to take multivitamins"*. Research shows that this is simply wrong. It has been clearly demonstrated that taking multivitamins improves useful immune response.[43][44] And this is important whether your T cells are 5 or 500.

One six-year study of 296 HIV(+) men completed at the University of California at Berkeley showed that there was a 31 percent reduction in the chance that the subjects would progress to a full-blown AIDS diagnosis if they just took a daily multivitamin. [18] *Doesn't this make it seem like everyone in the world should take a good multivitamin?*

Vitamins Help Ritonavir Go Down

Dr. Jon Kaiser, Harvard dietician Charlie Smigelski, and Dr. Lark Lands assert that building health with dietary supplements can improve the tolerance and response to AIDS medications. At the 38th ICAAC Conference (Abstract A-75) Gatti reported that of people taking Ritonavir, those with pre-existing nutrient deficiencies (Vitamins C, E, B12, folic acid, beta carotene), were over twice as likely (58% Vs 27%) to be unable to tolerate Ritonavir; those who took vitamin supplements were over twice as likely to respond to Ritonavir (69% Vs 32%); and the vitamin-takers had less Ritonavir-induced nausea, vomiting and diarrhea.

Vitamins, Minerals, and Antioxidants with Muscle

Numerous studies show that optimal intake of specific vitamins or nutrients correlate with your best survival. Do not settle for low-dosage, Centrum-type vitamin or nutrient levels. Centrum does not even contain the RDA of all the essential vitamins and minerals, and the RDA is barely adequate for healthy people who have no health problems. Even then it is not optimal; the RDA will only supply a fraction of what you need. Get multivitamins with some muscle — they will help you stay alive and healthy.

Complete Daily Vitamins

For years I have recommended my father's very high-potency daily vitamin formula called the SuperNutrition Opti-Pack (complete daily vitamins, minerals, and antioxidants) as the most powerful and most cost effective foundation for a daily nutrient program. However, the newest SuperNutrition formula called The Super Blend may be even better with even more antioxidants than the Opti-Pack. I attest that these two formulas are the *best multivitamin values in the world,* per penny per milligram. This is not just hype; this can be verified by adding up the costs of the nutrients they contain and comparing them to other multi-vitamin formulas. To get charts that compare them to other popular formulas, call 1-800-262-2116 or 1-415-641-0212. Both formulas have superior levels of many of the nutrients I suggest (see below), along with generous amounts of antioxidants. There are a number of other great vitamin formulas on the market that can serve the HIV(+) person well; the Jarrow Pack and the AMNI Added Protection lll are two of the best. But no other formula gives you as much for your money as the Opti-Pack or the Super Blend.

It is important to emphasize that some of the multivitamin products that are marketed to the HIV community give you relatively small doses of very important nutrients, yet cost a lot more per milligram than the Opti-Pack, the Super Blend, the Jarrow Pack, or the AMNI Added Protection lll. The Opti-Pack and the Super Blend are available at buyer's clubs and health food stores; call 1-800-262-2116 for more information.

Vitamin Safety

While spokespeople from organizations with questionable agendas, including the United States Food and Drug Administration, have made erroneous statements that vitamins can be "as dangerous as drugs," just a little bit of research proves that this is not true. For instance, the first eight annual reports of the American Association of Poison Control Centers, which collected statistics from issues of the American Journal of Emergency Medicine, show that during the first 10-year reporting period of the 72 poison control stations there was no documentation of a death being caused by a vitamin, but there were 2,556 deaths attributed to over-the-counter medicines like aspirin, and more than 1,000,000 deaths from prescription drugs during the same time period. *Vitamins will never be as dangerous as drugs.*

Nutrient Tests

For optimal effects on improving your health while reducing any potential for negative effects caused by having too much of a given nutrient, ask your doctor to test the nutrient levels in your body. These tests include the comprehensive mineral analysis from Balco Labs (800-777-7122), or the vitamin analysis from Spectracell Labs (800-227-5227). Ask your doctor about these and other nutrient analysis tests. Taking them will help you know what vitamins and minerals you need to take in higher amounts and help you determine what is safe for you. While it might seem like a good idea to take high levels of all the nutrients because they are generally very safe, you might have an unusual problem with a specific nutrient. For instance, one HIV(+) man who has suffered from neuropathy found that his body was storing very high levels of vitamin B6. While vitamin B6 supplementation can help to reduce neuropathy, having too much of it can promote neuropathy. Supplementing with the nutrients that will help to correct deficiencies can decrease your chances of suffering from infections caused by a weakened immune system, but it is important to determine if there are any nutrients that you shouldn't take.

Basic Daily Vitamin and Nutrient Plan

This is a quick-look plan for a simple, effective dietary supplement program for the person who is on a budget but wants to cover a very broad range of some of the most important nutrients.

These nutrients should be taken three times per day.

Complete multi-vitamin - 25 to 50 mg B-complex including vitamin B6 with each meal.

Complete multi-mineral — the daily total equals 1000 mg calcium, 600 mg magnesium, 200 mcg selenium, 200 mcg chromium, 30 mg zinc, with all the other minerals.

Antioxidants — 1,000 to 2,000 mg of vitamin C and 400 IU of vitamin E per meal.

N-acetyl cysteine - 500 mg per meal.

Acidophilus as a powder or capsules, as the label indicates.

Glutamine — With each meal, 1 teaspoon for basic maintenance up to 1 heaping tablespoon when there is weight loss or illness.

EPA fish oil capsules — 2 per meal.

Alpha lipoic acid — 50 to 100 mg per meal.

More Than Once A Day

Notice that this plan says "with each meal." Even if you can not be disciplined enough to take your daily nutrients three times per day, try to divide the total amount and take them twice per day. It is important to spread your nutrients out throughout the day rather than take them all at one meal because most nutrients only stay in the blood for a few hours. So try to take them in divided doses to keep blood levels relatively constant for optimal effect.

Take Vitamins With Meals

Taking most nutrients after you eat some food improves absorption for two reason; first, smelling food, and chewing and eating stimulate the secretion of gastric juices and enzymes that improve digestion and absorption. Second, having some food mass in your gastro-intestinal system slows the movement of the nutrients down so that they do not pass through rapidly without being broken down.

An Optimal Plan

You can go further with a daily nutrient program that I consider to be more optimal if your budget allows. Here are the optimal daily doses of vitamins, minerals, and other supplements I recommend for people with HIV. The doses may be high relative to the recommendations of people who are more conservative than I, but the published medical literature shows that the doses I suggest are not generally considered to be toxic, and may be much more beneficial than lower doses for HIV(+) people. Many of these nutrients are contained in sufficient levels in the SuperNutrition Opti-Pack and the Super Blend, but for optimal health it may be wise to use one of these vitamin formulas as a foundation and add booster levels of some of the most important nutrients.

The *italicized statements* delineate the nutrients known to reduce HIV progression and increase the potential for survival. Items are not listed in order of importance.

Again, the nutrients that should be taken three times per day.

Vitamins

1. **The B complex** — 50 to 100 mg with each meal three times per day. Necessary for energy metabolism, several B vitamins have been correlated to *increased survival*.

2. **Vitamin B6** — 50 to 100 mg three times per day should be included in your B-complex supplement. B6 is being used to treat neuropathy in doses up to 400 mg per day by nutritionally-oriented Dr. Jon Kaiser of San Francisco. Too much B6 can cause neuropathy, so it is wise to have your B6 status measured before high dose supplementation. B6 supplementation can reduce

elevated levels of the toxic amino acid metabolite called homocysteine,[100] so B6 supplementation may have a role in reducing the potential for cardiovascular disease[74] that can be caused by protease inhibitors. One HIV study showed that supplementation of 20 to 25 mg per day produced an improved CD4 to CD8 ratio, and an *average 121-point increase in CD4 T-cell counts over 6 months.*[71] B6 supplementation has also been associated with reduced depression[73] *and improved survival.*[72]

Peripheral Neuropathy

While vitamin B6 and the nutrients calcium, magnesium, alpha lipoic acid and acetyl-l-carnitine can each help neuropathy, several Western medical doctors and nurses credibly assert that the most effective treatment for neuropathy is acupuncture. We also have credible reports that one tablespoon of cod liver oil twice per day stops neuropathy for some individuals.

---

3. **Vitamin B12** — 100 to 300 mcg three times per day if taken orally. However, I believe that most HIV(+) people should be given prescriptions so that you can give yourself B12 injections because absorption through the gut is often compromised in HIV(+) people. (Typical injection doses are 1,000 mcg once per month for healthy people, up to three times per week for people who are ill or highly progressed.) *Cellular B12 levels have been shown to be correlative with improved survival,*[20] *and increased CD4 T-cell counts.*[19] Additionally, B12 deficiency is correlated with decreased mental function in HIV,[40] so it may help AIDS-related dementia. And finally, B12 helps to reduce homocysteine levels in the blood,[70] so it is also one of the nutrients that can help to reduce the potential for cardiovascular disease.

4. **Folic acid** — 400 to 1,000 mcg three times per day. (I take 1,000 mcg three times per day.) Improves immune function, white and red blood cell counts, and protein metabolism. Folic acid is one of the most powerful nutrients to reduce homocysteine, so it too reduces the potential for cardiovascular disease.[27] [70] Folic acid also improves states of clinical depression.[26] If you take folic acid you should take vitamin B12, as folic acid can mask a B12 deficiency. It appears that there is a chance that folic acid supplementation over about 5,000 mcg per day may cause increased production of red blood cells, which can promote strokes. So consult with your doctor before any use of ultra high doses.

5. **Vitamin A** — A good general recommendation for HIV(+) people is 5,000 IU of vitamin A per day total, regardless of your beta carotene intake. Some people think that beta carotene can substitute for vitamin A, but vitamin A has distinct anti tumor value that beta carotene does not appear to deliver as well. *Optimal vitamin A status has been shown to improve chances of survival and correlate with higher CD4 T-cell counts.*[37] Vitamin A deficiency appears to increase the chance of mother to child transmission of HIV.[39] Vitamin A can be toxic to the liver in very high doses, so people with liver problems should consult with their doctor before increasing their vitamin A dosage. Optimal vitamin A status improves insulin sensitivity,[78] so vitamin A is a nutrient that might help reduce lipodystrophy. Vitamin A is also required for healthy testosterone metabolism,[102] and growth hormone production.[103]

6. **Vitamin C** — 1,000 to 3,000 mg three times per day for maintenance, and up to 20,000 mg per day when ill. Vitamin C has a bowel-tolerance level effect. This means that when you take more than the amount that your body needs, you will get gas and then maybe diarrhea. This is basically harmless. Many people find that they can take much more than their normal

bowel tolerance level when they are sick — without getting diarrhea, as the body appears to use it up at a higher rate during illness. To find the optimum dose when fighting illness, raise the amount you take until you get some gas, then back off a little to a lower dose that causes no problem.

7. **Vitamin E** — 200 to 800 IU three times per day. This important antioxidant vitamin is the best nutrient to reduce the potential for atherosclerosis caused by protease inhibitors because it inhibits the oxidation of blood cholesterol and triglycerides. If enough vitamin E is present in the blood, elevated cholesterol or triglycerides have much less chance of oxidizing and contributing to atherosclerosis. One new study reported that vitamin E supplementation improves T-cell response.[32] Another study showed a decrease in the catabolic cytokine IL-1 with 1200 IU of daily vitamin E.[33] *Studies show that vitamin E is one of the nutrients that is most correlative with reducing HIV progression to AIDS.*[32][38] Optimal vitamin E status also improves insulin sensitivity,[77] so vitamin E is a nutrient that might help reduce some lipodystrophy symptoms.

Vitamins C and E Reduce VIRAL LOAD

A placebo-controlled study of 49 subjects over 3 months using 1000 mg of vitamin C combined with 800 IU of vitamin E per day showed reduced oxidative stress, reduced plasma lipid oxidation, and a trend towards reduction in viral load (-0.45-log versus +0.5-log for placebo). The researchers said. *"This is worthy of larger clinical trials, especially in HIV(+) people who cannot afford new combination therapies."* [107] This has important implications for all HIV(+) people, but especially for people in Third World countries that cannot afford the expensive antiretroviral AIDS medications.

Minerals

1. **Calcium** — 300 mg or more three times per day. Take for strong bones, nerve health, and muscle growth itself. Calcium and magnesium are nutrients that Dr. Jon Kaiser recommends to prevent and treat neuropathy. Optimal calcium intake improves insulin sensitivity,[79] so calcium is another nutrient that might help reduce some lipodystrophy symptoms.

2. **Magnesium** — 200 mg or more three times per day. Necessary for bone, heart and nerve health, and muscle growth and strength. Also involved in healthy insulin metabolism, so magnesium supplementation likely reduces the potential for some lipodystrophy symptoms.

3. **Zinc** — 10 to 30 mg three times per day. Improves healing and immune function. While one poorly designed questionnaire-based study suggested that having too much zinc might decrease survival in HIV,[21] other studies show that; there is a correlation with low zinc status and an increase in bacterial infections;[22] that high dose zinc supplementation (200 mg per day) can reduce the incidence of the deadly lung infection called pneumocystis and candida infections, *and cause an increase in CD4 T cells* and body weight,[23] and *that low zinc status is associated with increased risk of death.*[24] While there is an upper limit to how much zinc is safe because it can interfere with selenium's beneficial antitumor and antiviral effects, after communicating with leading zinc researchers, I find that the potential safe upper dose limit for short term use appears to be approximately 150 mg per day. Zinc is required for healthy testosterone production,[104] and IGF-1 production.[105] Zinc is best taken alone before bedtime for optimal absorption.

Nutrition expert Dr. Richard Beach at the University of Miami says that many HIV(+) people need 75 or more mg of zinc per day, and Dr. Baum's study, as cited above, indicated 90 mg per day was needed to get adequate blood levels for many people.

While I would not suggest overloading with zinc, poor zinc absorption and increased need for zinc by HIV(+) people makes some level of zinc supplementation very important. (Note: an overload is not well defined, and is very individual.) If a person is ill or is highly progressed, it is possible that they will need as much as 90 to 200 mg of zinc per day. High-dose zinc is generally only advisable for short periods of time, though, and for specific reasons. Ask your doctor or a certified nutritionist or registered dietitian if you think you might need high doses of zinc, and show them this information because they may not be aware of it. Symptoms of zinc deficiency are poor sense of smell and taste, slow healing, poor quality skin and hair, and low neutrophil counts.

4. **Selenium** — 100 to 200 mcg three times per day. Works with vitamin E, and helps in the generation of glutathione, the body's critically important natural antioxidant. One HIV study found correlations between CD4 T-cell counts, selenium levels, and glutathione levels.[31] In a study of 125 HIV-infected men and women, Dr. Marianna Baum found that *patients with selenium deficiency were 19.9 times more likely to die of AIDS than patients with adequate selenium levels.* She theorizes that the link between selenium and mortality is due to selenium's antioxidant function or action in gene regulation that might actually affect the replication of HIV itself. *"In selenium deficiency the HIV virus reproduces faster,"* she said.[24]

5. **Copper** — 2 mg. Necessary for healing, and helps form super oxide dismutase (SOD), an important antioxidant enzyme in the body. If you are taking high dose zinc (more than 40 mg) you may need to take more than 2 mg of copper, as high dose zinc can cause a copper deficiency. Copper is critical to immune health and antioxidant production in the body. Ask your doctor to test for zinc and copper deficiencies.

6. **Chromium** — 300 mcg three times per day. Chromium improved insulin sensitivity 40 percent in a study with diabetics without toxicity at 1000 mcg per day,[28] so chromium is another nutrient that might help reduce some lipodystrophy symptoms. (Chromium's potentially toxic dose is considered to be about 70,000 mcg per day according to the U.S. Environmental Protection Agency.)

7. **Iron** — 18 to 50 mg. A 6-year University of California at Berkeley study showed that iron intake was *highly correlative with reducing progression of HIV to full-blown AIDS,* and 54 mg per day from food and supplements appeared to be about twice as good as 36 mg to reduce HIV progression.[18] Iron is very poorly absorbed in general, so supplementation can be very important for people who are anemic and have very low energy. Iron is necessary for the production of carnitine in the body, the health of the red blood cells, immune health, the body's ability to fight bacteria, and energy production.

Iron is an essential nutrient and the body utilizes iron for optimal health properly when oxidative activity in the body is under control because there are an abundance of antioxidants derived from a healthy diet and dietary supplements. Optimal iron status is required for overall health in early HIV, however, there is a potential for iron overload in HIV, especially in the more advanced stages,[29] or when antioxidant status in the body is compromised, or when there is insulin resistance.[101] Iron overload can increase the potential for immune problems and increased infections, so it is advisable to ask your doctor to test and monitor your iron level.

The standard iron storage test called *serum ferritin* may not accurately reflect excess iron stored in the liver, heart, bone marrow, etc., according to Sharon McDonnell, MD, MPH, of the Centers for Disease Control. She says that testing for *transferrin saturation* provides a more accurate indication of this kind of stored iron, especially if it is elevated in more than one test.

For those of you who do include iron in their daily supplementation, there is one form of iron that is considered to be basically nontoxic, even at doses in the thousands of milligrams. This form is called *iron carbonyl*,[60] and it is the form of iron contained in the SuperNutrition and the AMNI vitamin formulas.

Vitamin E Keeps Iron Safe

Studies indicate that iron's potential for oxidative toxicity is greatly reduced by keeping your vitamin E status optimal, with one mouse study showing that high doses of vitamin E totally prevented the lethal dose of iron from killing the mice.[30] Protect your health; be sure that high dose vitamin E is part of your daily nutrient intake.

Special Antioxidants

1. **Beta carotene** and other carotenes like lycopene and lutein. I recommend 12,000 IU of beta carotene. *Optimal intake of beta carotene has been shown to increase CD4 T-cell counts and the chances of survival in HIV.*[21]

2. **Sulfur antioxidant amino acids — Methionine** at 300 to 500 mg three times per day. Methionine is a precursor that converts to carnitine in the body. **N-acetyl**

cysteine (NAC) 500 to 1,000 mg three times per day. The common cysteine form **L-cysteine** can also be taken, and for some purposes, like reducing alcohol toxicity, it may be slightly superior to NAC,[60] but NAC is preferred overall for HIV because NAC appears to increase glutathione production more efficiently.[41] [42] While I have heard people say that L-cysteine can be "toxic", L-cysteine is not toxic if you keep it in its reduced state by taking in plenty of extra vitamin C. Just be sure to take about three times as much vitamin C as L-cysteine.

The Herzenberg study showed that high-dose NAC intake (3,200 to 8,000 mg per day) correlated with increased survival.[35] It is likely that a lower dose of NAC (1,200 to 2,400 mg) would work just as well if L-glutamine is taken also because either of them alone will increase glutathione production. (See glutamine below.) I suggest a dose of one teaspoon of the powdered form of glutamine one to three times per day for this purpose.

Taking alpha lipoic acid with NAC would also logically increase the effect of NAC, so that a moderate dose of NAC (2,000 mg) may work as well as a high dose (3,000 to 8,000 mg). (See ALA information below.)

A recent six month study of 262 HIV(-) men and women showed that taking only 600 mg of NAC per day helped the immune system so much that the NAC users suffered from the flu only one third as much as those who did not take NAC.[49] Everyone in the world would probably be healthier if we all took NAC.

I emphasize that taking NAC can raise glutathione levels in the body, but taking glutathione itself orally does not, as it is destroyed very quickly after ingestion. Also note that the Herzenberg study states: *"the unnecessary or excessive use of acetaminophen (Tylenol), alco-*

hol, or other drugs known to deplete glutathione should be avoided by HIV-infected individuals." While an occasional beer or wine may not present that much problem to some people, ideally HIV(+) people would avoid alcohol, especially if they are using liver toxic medications.

3. **Alpha lipoic acid** (ALA) — 100 to 300 mg three times per day. *ALA is perhaps the most important antioxidant for HIV(+) people to take.* It appears to be a nutrient that will be shown to be very effective for reducing damage to the liver for people who are taking liver toxic medications. It is known that ALA helps in the production and recycling of the critically important cellular antioxidant glutathione,[34] so taking ALA causes the glutathione level in the blood to increase. Alpha lipoic acid also may have the potential to benefit those people who have peripheral neuropathy, as it has been shown to be beneficial to neuropathy caused by diabetes.[36] Finally, it also improves insulin sensitivity, so it also may help to reduce some lipodystrophy symptoms.

4. **Coenzyme Q10** (CoQ10) — 30 to 100 mg three times per day with meals. A super antioxidant and important for immune function, energy metabolism, and heart health. Some HIV(+) people report a tremendous improvement in energy with high dose CoQ10 (300mg per day).

Specialty Supplements

1. **Omega-3 and omega-6 fatty acids** — Alpha linolenic acid (ALA), and linoleic acid (LA) become EPA (omega-3) and GLA (omega-6) in the body. Note, many HIV(+) people and some HIV(-) people are deficient in the enzymes in the body that convert ALA and LA into the finished fatty acids, which become prostaglandins in the body. *Proper prostaglandin function*

is necessary for healthy cellular immune function. While one popular source of GLA (omega-6) is evening primrose oil, GLA from borage is more cost effective. The best source of EPA (omega-3) is marine lipids from cold water fish oil capsules. You can also get these by eating fish like salmon, sardines, and tuna.

Flax oil has both omega-3 and omega-6 in a good balance that favors omega-3. As noted before, most people do not get enough omega-3 from their diet, but get relatively too much omega-6. Omega-6 tends to increase inflammatory activity in the body when there is not enough omega-3, which is anti-inflammatory. Too much omega-6 is not good for HIV. Try to get more omega-3, but you do need both in balance.

A deficiency of either essential fatty acid could increase AIDS progression, as they are both necessary for healthy, balanced immune function. Get these fatty acids as fresh as possible, as they are delicate and oxidize easily. Oxidized fats are bad for the immune system.

GLA (from borage) is taken as one capsule two times per day. EPA is taken as two capsules three times per day with meals. Or take one tablespoon of fresh refrigerated flax oil two times per day.

Flax oil appears to cause allergic reactions in some people. If you use flax oil, make sure it is fresh, because it is a highly perishable, easily oxidizing oil. It should be kept in the refrigerator, and if it starts to taste bitter, the fatty acids are beginning to go rancid and turn to trans fatty acids, so throw it out and get a fresh bottle. I recommend that you buy small bottles for this reason.

2. **Carnitine** — 1,000 to 2,000 mg three times per day. Or **acetyl-L-carnitine**, a more efficiently absorbed version of carnitine, at 500 to 1,000 mg three times per

day. The prescription version of carnitine called Carnitor is covered by insurance, so you can save money if you can get your doctor to prescribe it. Carnitine helps reduce triglyceride levels in the blood and is necessary to carry fats into the mitochondria of the cell to be burned for energy. Hypertriglyceridemia (elevated triglycerides), and cellular energy metabolism problems are common in HIV and natural production of the body's carnitine is frequently lower than normal, so everyone who is HIV-positive could probably benefit from taking supplemental carnitine.[45] The decrease in triglycerides can help reduce the potential for atherosclerosis that is being associated with protease inhibitor use. Low carnitine can also contribute to the loss of muscle tissue. Carnitine is also one of the nutrients that is known to help reduce neuropathy and acetyl-L-carnitine deficiency is associated with the peripheral neuropathy that is caused by neurotoxic nucleoside analogs (ddI, ddC, d4T).[75 76] Acetyl-L-carnitine can reduce dementia in Alzheimer's patients.[46] Maybe it will be shown to help with AIDS-related dementia, too. And finally, a recent study showed that high dose (6,000 mg/day) carnitine infusions increased CD4 T-cell counts.[80]

3. **Acidophilus** — Lactobacillus acidophilus and the other friendly bacteria supplements are taken to increase the healthy intestinal bacteria. They help to manufacture some vitamins, and are critical to the health of the intestines, as they keep the various bacteria in the intestines, like candida albicans, in check. Acidophilus supplementation can help people who have gas and diarrhea. Antibiotics kill acidophilus, so after you have used antibiotics you should take acidophilus every day for a week or so to replenish the acidophilus in your intestines.

One study showed that acidophilus increased the absorption of iron and improved hemoglobin generation, so it appeared to help the body use iron so it can build the red blood cells better.[47]

Acidophilus is best bought in dry form and kept cold. There are lab reports that show little to no live acidophilus in several of the liquid products, so it is advisable you to buy it in capsules or, for the best savings, as a powder.

4. **Digestive Aids** — For protein digestion take pancreatin, pepsin, betaine HCL, and glutamic acid HCL. Hydrochloric acid (HCL) is deficient in the stomach of many HIV(+) people. I know wasting HIV(+) people who have chronic diarrhea who take as much as 9 grams of betaine or glutamic acid or a combination of both of them with protein meals and enjoy a great reduction in diarrhea. If you produce insufficient gastric acid you will be more prone to developing myobacterium avium complex (MAC) and cytomegalovirus (CMV) in the gut, as lower acid levels in the stomach allow microbes to pass into the gut.

For fat digestions take lipase, a fat-digesting enzyme. Multiple enzyme products like Megazyme by Enzymatic Therapy or Jarrowzyme with protease (for protein), lipase (for fat), and amylase (for carbohydrates), may help improve digestion a lot. Enzymatic Therapy's Protazyme is specific for protein digestion.

Chew your food thoroughly. Chewing increases your internal enzyme production.

5. **Glandulars — Andrenal, Pituitary, Liver, Thymus** — Glandulars feed the organs in the body. Glandulars that may be beneficial include adrenal, thymus, pituitary, liver, and hypothalamus. Glandulars

are controversial — mainstream Western medicine does not think they provide any benefit. I consider this opinion to be a result of a misunderstanding of the possible mechanisms of action. Personal experience causes me to believe glandulars do have an effect. However, they are not a highly profitable supplement, so no company will spend money studying them. We may never see good-quality data that document any potential effect. However, some older publications do infer a benefit. For instance, an old article in the Lancet in 1952 showed that liver supplementation radically improved stamina and endurance in lab animals. Old-time boxing trainers know this and tell boxers to eat liver for endurance. It works very well. It is also the best source of supplemental iron, as the iron in it called heme iron absorbs about 10 times better than what is found in dietary supplements. (See the information on iron above.)

A new supplement called BioThymic Protein A is an example of a glandular extract that is reported to improve thymus function and immune function. BioThymic Protein A is available from natural foods stores and HIV-buyer's clubs.

An Herbal Extract

Standardized (Milk Thistle) Extract (silymarin herb) — this important herbal extract is a potent liver protector that appears to improve protein synthesis in the liver that can help regenerate damaged liver tissue.[62-64] Recommended dose: 150 mg to 300 mg three times per day. Only buy standardized silymarin extract. As with many herbs, the active ingredients in the herb must be extracted to maximize effectiveness. Raw powdered silymarin in capsules does not do the job. As noted in the Lipodystrophy chapter, silymarin can improve insulin sensitivity, too.

An Important Amino Acid

Glutamine — 4 grams (1 heaping teaspoon) three times per day for health maintenance, or 12 grams (1 heaping tablespoon) three times per day when ill, losing weight or to build muscle. Do not bother with glutamine in capsules as you need higher doses than the capsules can give you.

Glutamine is the one dietary supplement that is truly anabolic and anticatabolic for muscle tissue. Studies show that it can not only increase muscle protein synthesis (anabolism),[53] but decrease breakdown (catabolism) of muscle tissue.[54] L-glutamine is essential for the health of the intestinal immune cells called gut associated lymphoid tissue (GALT).[55] *Glutamine is also necessary for the generation and function of T cells.*[56 57] And, finally, it is one of the very best supplements to increase production of the liver's detoxifying enzyme called glutathione when the liver is challenged by liver-toxic medications.[52] As noted before, it is likely that it is even more effective in improving glutathione when combined with 1,200 to 2,400 mg of N-acetyl cysteine per day.

Those who have diarrhea will likely experience a tremendous reduction in diarrhea by supplementing with 12 grams of glutamine three times per day when diarrhea occurs, then maintaining a dose of 12 or more grams per day. This is because glutamine is critically important for the regeneration of the digestive system intestinal mucous membranes.[58] A study by Prang, that was presented at the International Conference on AIDS Wasting in November of 1997, showed that wasting HIV patients who were given 30 to 40 grams of glutamine per day stopped losing weight and started gaining weight. Additionally, diarrhea stopped in the two patients in the study who had chronic diarrhea.[59] See the reprint of the abstract that follows.

Glutamine Doses Needed

How much L-glutamine should an HIV(+) person use? Many people with diarrhea will need 30 to 50 grams per day for anywhere from a few weeks to several months while intestinal tissue repair is occurring. After that, a maintenance dose might be about 12 grams per day. Look for the second book about glutamine by Dr. Judy Shabert for detailed information. With little potential for toxicity, glutamine presents several tremendously important benefits to HIV(+) individuals. Bulk powdered glutamine can be purchased through several of the HIV-buyer's clubs by the kilogram at an affordable price.

Anabolic Steroids Can Enhance Glutamine Uptake

Another potential benefit of appropriate anabolic steroid therapy is the improvement in nutrient uptake that they appear to effect. One study showed that nandrolone decanoate (Deca Durabolin) doubled glutamine and tripled alanine uptake in the gut after surgery.[7]

L-Glutamine Promotes Gain in Weight and Body Cell Mass in Patients with AIDS
by E. Prang, LCN, C. Stoltz, RD, and J. Shabert, MD, MPH, RD

Weight loss commonly occurs with AIDS, and appetite stimulants and anabolic agents have been utilized in an attempt to reverse this catabolic state. Nutritional interventions, which enhance caloric intake are generally associated with fat and water gain, not enhancement of lean tissue. We evaluated the effect of administering the amino acid L-glutamine to 10 subjects (9 males, 1 female) with non-IV drug related HIV infections. All subjects had weight loss (body weight 90 percent of ideal) and two had diarrhea (pasty or liquid stool 4 times per day). All received 30-40 grams of L-glutamine per day in divided doses (Cambridge Nutraceuticals, Boston, MA) for at least 12 weeks in this phase 1 open-label trial. Following baseline studies, the patients were evaluated monthly; bodyweight, and bioelectrical impedance assessment were performed (RJL Systems, Clinton, MI). Routine chemistries and hematology obtained during this time were reviewed. The average values for the group are shown in the table below.

No adverse effects were noted. Both subjects with diarrhea had complete resolution of this symptom during the study. Six of the patients continued an additional 6 months of L-glutamine supplementation and gained an additional 0.8 kg over this time period.

L-glutamine, a conditionally essential amino acid, can replete body protein in depleted AIDS patients. The increase in intracellular water which occurs signals protein anabolism as reflected by the increase in body cell mass. Randomized blinded trials are now indicated to confirm these findings, which demonstrate that gain in functioning protein-containing tissue can be achieved by providing this low cost amino acid supplement to AIDS patients.

Comment: Note that the glutamine not only stopped weight loss, but stopped diarrhea in the two subjects who had it.

N = 10	Before	After	P value by paired t-test
Weight (kg)	73.0	75.5	0.02
Body cell mass (L)	29.5	30.5	0.037
Total body water (L)	44.1	45.3	0.021
Intracellular Water (L)	26.9	27.8	0.039
Extracellular Water (L)	17.2	17.5	NS
Phase angle	6.5	6.8	0.154

Over-the-Counter Hormones

DHEA (Dehydroepiandrosterone)

I recommend the use of a supplement available in health food stores, called DHEA, for continuous replacement supplementation for those who test as having low DHEA production, measured as DHEA-S in blood tests.

DHEA is an adrenal steroid and precursor to testosterone that causes a significant increase in testosterone production in women. For men, the studies show no significant effect on testosterone production.[82][83] Women also typically experience a more profound improvement in feelings of well-being than men, as DHEA can have a powerful antidepressive effect.[84]

DHEA has also been to shown to have potential as an antitumor/anticancer agent,[85] and it has anti-HIV effects in vitro.[86] One study showed that DHEA levels decreased in HIV(+) people when CD4 T cells were below 500.[92] Most recently, data are accumulating that show that DHEA's potential beneficial effects against HIV may be caused by a reduction in tumor necrosis factor-a,[87] and an interference with NF-kappa B activation.[88] This means that DHEA replacement supplementation, when shown to be appropriate by lab tests, could possibly slow the progression of HIV disease.[89]

If you are getting the idea that I am proposing that all HIV(+) people should strongly consider supplementing with DHEA, you are right. I also caution that you should have DHEA tests done and *work with your doctor* to find an optimal replacement dose that is specific for you.

Although studies have not yet shown what blood levels are truly optimal for males and females, most doctors test to find a dosage that brings a person into the range that a 25 to 30 year-old healthy person would have. (Again, dosage is something to work on with your doctor.) If a person suffers from low energy, poor mood, or symptoms typical of a severe androgen hormone deficiency, they may find that they need to use DHEA for several weeks before blood levels reach optimum.[83]

I also have feedback from several men, having come off steroid cycles and crashed a few weeks after stopping a cycle, who report experiencing an immediate improvement in state of mind and overall energy level with DHEA supplementation. While HIV-negative men over 40 years of age would tend to use DHEA at a dosage of around 50 mg per day, HIV(+) men appear to sometimes need higher daily doses, from 100 mg to even 400 mg.

Special Consideration — Women

I have seen women who tested as having both low DHEA and low testosterone experience optimal elevations of both by supplementing with DHEA alone. I have also seen women try testosterone replacement creams and feel very uncomfortable. Often, when they switch to DHEA their DHEA and testosterone levels both increase and they feel great. Women should consider that DHEA supplementation by itself may be all they need. Appropriate daily doses for women appear to be between 10 and 100 mg. Women should be especially careful in finding an appropriate dose, as DHEA can cause virilizing effects in women. The first manifestations of virilization from excessive dosing in women are usually oily skin, acne, and/or dark peach fuzz. If any of these are detected, work with your doctor to decrease your dosage or stop any use. These symptoms usually reverse if DHEA supplementation is stopped immediately.

Cautions

I caution men with prostate problems to only implement DHEA under the supervision of your doctor, as the available data suggest that, while DHEA may have some anticancer effects,[85] it might also promote prostate cancer.[90] While DHEA may inhibit certain types of breast cancer,[91] women with signs of early-stage breast cancer should only use DHEA under a doctor's supervision.

All HIV(+) males and females should only use DHEA under your doctor's supervision. It can be quite valuable for HIV(+) people, but it *is* a hormone and ideally its use should be monitored.

Bodybuilding Supplements and DHEA

DHEA has been appearing in "kitchen sink" bodybuilding formulas mixed with several other purported testosterone boosters. DHEA is not necessarily a useful addition to these kinds of formulas, as it actually might decrease the effectiveness of products like androstenedione, which is discussed below. This is because DHEA competes for an enzyme (17-beta hydroxysteroid dehydrogenase) that converts androstenedione to testosterone, and so it might decrease the net amount of testosterone produced by this process. It also might cause more estrogen production and estrogenic activity because of its potential to convert to 5-androstenediol.

Androstenedione and Androstenediol

I have also investigated the new pro-hormone products that are sold over the counter at health food stores and some of the buyer's clubs called androstenedione (ADN) and 4-androstenediol (4-ADL). Pro-hormones are immediate testosterone precursors that are one step closer to testosterone than DHEA. Each of them has a much more profound effect on testosterone production than DHEA for women *and* men. Androstenedione decline has been correlated to a decline in CD4 T cells in HIV,[92] so it is remotely possible that androstenedione supplementation might be beneficial to immune metabolism but this is not known. HIV(+) men are reporting good effects on energy and libido when taking these pro-hormones at a dosage of 50 to 100 mg two to three times per day, but there are no data that are specific to HIV, or data that confirms that they actually affect muscle growth or what dosing might actually promote muscle growth. Pro-hormones have the potential to increase hair loss and cause other side effects that are characteristic of testosterone, so they should be viewed as another way to increase testosterone, and not toys. I do not have any data

on safe use for women, and they have potential to cause significant virilizing side effects to women, so I caution against any use by women.

ADs do not require functional testes because they increase testosterone by converting primarily in the liver. This means that they will not help men regain their normal testicular testosterone production after they have used anabolic steroids.

It is believed that the potential value of pro-hormones for HIV(+) men in the forms they are currently available in is not as a true testosterone replacement therapy, but only as a quick boost tonic to be used to help improve feelings of quality-of-life and libido. They also may have a role for periods of time between steroid cycles to improve energy, mood and libido, and perhaps help maintain lean body mass.

Logically, for pro-hormones to increase muscle growth by increasing testosterone, the increase in testosterone would have to be maintained a majority of the time, as testosterone's anabolic cellular effects take place as a succession of events over several days. An AD product that does not have some time-release mechanism, or is not taken several times per day, may have a quick effect on libido or drive, because some of the neurochemical effects of testosterone can happen in minutes,[93][94] but their effects on muscle growth, which take place as a series of biochemical activities that happen over a period of days, would be compromised if they were only taken once per day.

AD products that contain no agent to slow their release generally deliver a quick peak blood level within the first 30 to 90 minutes and then dissipate within about three to four hours. Several researchers have verified this effect by doing blood tests. AD products that are marketed as time-released are beginning to be sold, and I welcome this as an improvement that may make this product more effective, if the makers really do use a quality time-release method.

Since time-release is somewhat expensive, be skeptical when a company says that it has a time-release product. Hopefully, some company will eventually make a time-released AD product that can be considered to be medical grade.

I also have reports of a few doctors prescribing ADs to HIV(+) males and hope that there will be controlled studies with either 4-androstenediol or androstenedione or both of these pro-hormones someday.

Comparing Androstenedione and Androstenediol

Blood tests I have done and others' blood tests confirm that 4-ADL does appear to raise testosterone more than ADN.

5-Androstenediol

Another pro-hormone called 5-androstenediol (5-AD) is also being sold by bodybuilding shops, health food stores, and some of the buyer's clubs. 5-AD should convert to testosterone at a lesser rate than 4-ADL, and it has intrinsic estrogenic activity, so it is much less desirable than 4-ADL. Because of its estrogenic effects it also appears that it has more potential to promote enlargement of the prostate. I recommend against its use.

Nor-Androstenedione/diol

Nor-androstenedione or nor-androstenediol convert to nandrolone in the body and may produce an anabolic effect with less potential for side effects like hair loss, and acne than the ADs. More than likely with high doses, though, any anabolic effect of the nors would be about the same as the similar AD product, but 4-androstenediol may increase physical strength somewhat more, just as testosterone may produce more strength increases than nandrolone once a given blood level is reached.[95]

With proper use of these over-the-counter hormones it may be easier to maintain feelings of quality-of-life between steroid cycles. They are not, at this time however, substitutes for appropriate testosterone replacement therapy. Again, if you decide to supplement with these hormone products, consider working with your doctor, and have them monitor you so that you can learn about any actual positive or negative effects.

Other Dietary Supplements

The following dietary supplements are sold as bodybuilding supplements. Bodybuilding supplements tend to be the most hyped, dishonestly marketed products in the world of dietary supplements, so skepticism is warranted.

Chrysin

Is chrysin effective as an anti-estrogen at reasonable doses? Is it a natural substitute for Arimidex or Nolvadex? Synthetic chemist Patrick Arnold, the man who introduced chrysin to the supplement market has his doubts. Since I have seen no lab tests that confirm that it works, so do I. I suggest that any manufacturer who makes a chrysin product consider doing appropriate lab tests to verify its effects. Whatever company does publish legitimate lab work to confirm a beneficial effect will be far ahead of the pack of wildcat companies who have no credible data to support the claims that are being made.

Tribulus

Does the herb tribulus terrestris increase testosterone? The one study that asserts this is suspect, so I need more independent data to believe it. It is known to be a Middle European adaptogenic tonic herb, and elite Eastern Bloc athletes do use it for improved recovery, but this does not mean it increases testosterone. Tribulus is appearing in "kitchen sink" bodybuilding formulas with androstenedione. If tribulus does in fact, cause the testes to produce testosterone, it still would likely do nothing to promote androstenedione's conversion to testosterone, as androstenedione converts primarily in the liver, not the testes. Be wary of products like these if you have a real medical need to increase testosterone, as they probably will not deliver what you need.

Lysophosphatidyl Choline

I advise against the use of androstenedione products (or any products) that contain lysophosphatidyl choline (LPC). It is also known as lysolecithin and Plasmologen, which is being marketed in bodybuilding stores as an absorption aid. LPC can increase intestinal (and other) cell-wall permeability, but intestinal cell walls have very tightly controlled permeability for protective reasons — to keep things out of the body *and* in the body. Solid data in the medical literature verify that LPC has the potential to seriously inflame and injure intestinal cells.[96][97] I have received reports of people experiencing chronic colitis after the use of LPC, and it definitely has the potential to promote food allergies, cardiovascular problems,[98] and other problems related to cellular inflammation.

Creatine Monohydrate

Creatine is perhaps the best supplement available for quick muscular cosmetic effects and strength improvement for both males and females. With creatine usage, muscles become fuller looking in a very short time, and the power of the muscles is enhanced. Dosing of creatine starts with a loading phase, where 30 grams per day is taken for the first five to seven days, then a maintenance dose of 3 to 5 grams is generally recommended. The truth is 10 grams per day for maintenance seems to work much better over the long run. It may be true that creatine use actually promotes biochemical changes in protein metabolism that affect muscle growth, but this is not proven yet. It does fill the muscle cells with fluid, which is called "cell volumizing," and it does enhance the body's cellular ATP production, which can result in increased strength and power.

Most people find that when they stop continuous use of creatine, they lose water and weight quickly. Still, it can be a useful adjunct to a weight-training program and can be used effectively during or between steroid cycles to maintain and improve muscular strength.

Caution: Some PoWeR clients have complained about becoming very bloated with creatine. This may be because of a unique problem when creatine is used with some of the kidney-burdening AIDS medications, like Crixivan. Additionally, those who have sensitive gastrointestinal tracts should use creatine with caution as it can cause diarrhea in some people.

Results of the 60 Day SAINTS Program

I started this chapter by talking about my father's orthomolecular nutrition study undertaken before the introduction of protease inhibitors, so I will finish with a summation of that two-month study. People on an orthmolecular allergy-free diet that was determined for each individual and taking only a part of the supplements I discuss in this chapter experienced the following:

1. Although most of the people experienced a slight increase in CD4 and CD8 T cells, the average of the changes was not large enough to be called statistically significant. Feelings of quality-of-life improved a lot, but did not seem to correlate with T cell changes. (No testosterone or anabolic hormones were used.)

2. Initially people experienced an increase in diarrhea, probably because of the introduction of more fiber and fluids from the addition of more vegetables to their diet. However, by the end of the study the subjects reported an average 75 percent reduction in diarrhea, probably because of a reduction in food allergies, and an increase in the general health of their gastrointestinal systems. Note: The subjects did not take high doses of glutamine, which can reduce diarrhea even more.

3. Red blood cell values improved for most people. Mean corpuscular volume, hematocrit, and hemoglobin values increased (hemoglobin helps to deliver more oxygen

to the cells in your body). This is especially important for overall energy and every aspect of healthy metabolism, including setting the stage for best muscle growth.

4. Without an exercise program, their grip-strength, a measure of vitality, increased significantly.

5. People subjectively felt more energetic, and more upbeat, with less general symptoms.

6. Libido increased. Sometimes, not always, libido means an increase in natural testosterone production, free testosterone, or the body's response to its testosterone, however testosterone was not measured. It may also might mean healthier brain chemistry, perhaps via changes in dopamine or serotonin, but this is only speculation.

Conclusions

1. Orthomolecular nutrition can improve digestion and reduce AIDS-related diarrhea.

2. It can also help your body build healthier red blood cells. This is important for building lean tissue, improving overall health, and giving you the energy to exercise.

3. Orthomolecular nutrition can improve grip-strength, feelings of energy, well-being, and libido, with a reduction in general symptoms of illness.

4. While no significant increase in T cells was found in this short study, it would be interesting to do a longer study, perhaps six or twelve months in duration, because many other long-term studies, like the six-year University of California Abrams study, do show that the intake of various nutrients supports healthy T-cell counts, and a reduction in T cell decline.[18]

World's Lowest Cost Supplements — Specific Modules

You can obtain the most inexpensive dietary supplement program in the world (approximately 75 percent off retail prices) by taking part in my father's SAINTS nutrient study by calling (415) 641-0305. All you have to do is participate in the ongoing part of the study by submitting a copy of your lab work regularly.

Highly Recommended

To learn more about how specific nutrients can address health problems in HIV, get the *Nutritional Therapies* pamphlet from Houston Buyer's Club by calling 1 (800) 350-2392.

Pediatric AIDS: Approaches to Managing Wasting

by Michael Mooney

Anabolic Hormones

The use of oxandrolone and human growth hormone (GH) with male and female children has been investigated extensively for stunted-growth children. While work that specifically studies children with HIV/AIDS has not been completed yet, we assume that what has been determined to be effective for stunted-growth children is a good starting point for children with HIV/AIDS-related wasting.

These studies show that oxandrolone may be slightly more effective for growth than GH, but that the net of effect of the two is probably a little better than either alone.[1-3] If cost is a consideration, oxandrolone is the better choice, as a 25-kilogram male child would require roughly one tablet of oxandrolone per day at a cost of $3.75, or GH at a cost of approximately $27 per day.

Studies show that oxandrolone produces beneficial effects with as little as .05 mg per kg per day[4] and as much as .1 mg per kg per day,[2] with a female child likely requiring the smaller dose, and a male child the higher dose.

Oxandrolone has been found to produce slightly better results when combined with GH. The combination studies have shown benefit with GH employed at doses of .03 mg/kg per day,[4] and .03 mg three times per week.[2] (Any evidence of tumors would obviate the use of GH.) If the child begins to experience arthralgia (joint pain), the GH dose should be reduced somewhat to find an acceptable dose. This suggested dose for oxandrolone has been used safely with non-HIV stunted growth children, but it is possible, based on what often happens with adults, that the dose might have to be higher for a child who was highly catabolic and wasting.

No Estrogen-Producing Steroids

Use of anabolic steroids that convert to estrogen such as nandrolone or testosterone is not recommended, as estrogen will effect the closure of the epiphysis, so these steroids can stunt long-bone growth.

Protein Nutrition

Data suggests that protein requirements would likely be .75 to 1 gram of protein per pound of bodyweight per day for a person with AIDS (child or adult) who is losing lean body mass, as studies suggest that higher protein intake is beneficial when wasting is evident.[5] Again, the use of BIA is suggested to track any changes in body cell mass. The addition of cottage cheese to the diet will provide optimal quality protein for improvements in lean body mass.

The casein protein in cottage cheese has high levels of L-glutamine and is an optimal protein for improving nitrogen retention.[6]

As detailed in the chapter on orthomolecular nutrition, the whey protein supplement called Immunocal has been documented in several published studies to contains superior levels of glutamyl/cysteine, a precursor for glutathione production. These studies show that it does increase glutathione and improves immune health and lean body mass in HIV patients.[7][8]

The protein powder supplement called Optimune does not have significant published data as yet, but it appears to help reduce diarrhea because of its high immunoglobulin content, as immunoglobulins are known to decrease diarrhea by increasing antibody activity in the intestines.[9] (The protein contained in Optimune is used to induce passive immunity in calves, lambs, piglets in products sold in the veterinary industry.)

Dietary Supplements

Multivitamin supplementation and the use of the supplements suggested for adults in the chapter on orthomolecular would be applicable to children, but on a reduced scale that is consistent with the relative difference in body weight. All other dietary supplements that have been correlated to survival for adults are good for children too. Good supplements include a multi-vitamin/mineral supplement, N-acetyl cysteine, vitamin B-12, and essential fatty acids.

Suggested is the addition of L-glutamine to the child's dietary intake at a daily intake of .066 grams per pound of bodyweight if weight is stable. When wasting is evident, a study by Dr. Judy Shabert suggests that an effective dose could be as high as .2 grams per pound of body-weight. The daily dose should be divided and given 3 to 5 times per day. Powdered L-glutamine, available in cost-efficient bulk packaging, can be added to drinks or formula and has little taste. High dose L-glutamine use is being shown to stop wasting, increase lean body mass, and stop diarrhea in HIV. (See the reprint of Dr. Prang's glutamine study on page 111.)

Resistance Exercise

The child should be encouraged to exercise regularly, if possible, with some sort of resistance exercise modality like Thera-bands. Note: resistance training, not aerobic exercise, stimulates lean body mass growth. The exercise techniques described in this book for adults can generally be applied to children; the clinician can develop a child's individual program. Keep in mind that resistance exercise is best performed on alternate days so that there is enough time between sessions for adequate recovery and growth.

AIDS and Food Safety

HIV(+) individuals are greatly at risk of serious illness or death from food-borne infections. This problem can be handled, but you must take this issue very seriously and adopt several basic precautions.

Food-borne microorganisms cause tens of millions of cases of intestinal infection each year in the U.S. and around the world. Do not assume there will be no problems with this just because you are in the U.S. or another highly civilized country. For most healthy people, the distressful vomiting, abdominal cramps, and diarrhea are blessedly short-lived. But in people with weakened immunity, such as those with AIDS, symptoms are often severe and the infections are so difficult to treat that they can be fatal.

Bugs In The Food

The leading cause of bacterial diarrhea in the U.S., *Campylobacter jejuni* bacteria, induces up to 10 percent of all cases. Of the patients infected with this bacterium, about 1 in 1,000 dies. Half of the *C. jejuni* infections are associated with eating or handling chickens. Indeed, surveys show the bacterium contaminates anywhere from 20 to 100 percent of retail raw chickens. So cook your chicken well.

Other prime sources are raw, unpasteurized milk, nonchlorinated water, and red meat. Cross-contamination can occur from using the same cutting board to cut up raw chicken and then other foods without cleaning the board in between. Cross-contamination may also occur during storage of foods. This is a major pathway for *Salmonella* into the diet.

The *Salmonella* bacterium is perhaps the second-most-frequent bacterial offender, accounting for about 2 million to 4 million salmonellosis cases annually.

Individuals with AIDS, and possibly late-stage HIV infection, are at least 20 times more likely than other people to become infected with *Salmonella* and six times more likely to develop a blood infection, which can be life-threatening. In late-stage HIV disease, including AIDS, campylobacteriosis and salmonellosis tend to recur and are extremely difficult to treat.

Of the several types of *Listeria* bacteria, the only one responsible for illness in people is *Listeria monocytogenes*. Besides blood stream infection, listeriosis can lead to meningitis (inflammation of the membranes covering the brain and spinal cord) and encephalitis (inflammation of the brain).

The *Listeria* bacteria are found in unpasteurized milk; cold smoked fish, poultry and meat; undercooked poultry; and certain cheeses, particularly soft-ripened varieties such as Brie and Camembert. Even vegetables can carry *Listeria* and, once cut, support its growth. A quarter of the estimated 1600 listeriosis cases each year end in death. AIDS patients are 200 to 300 times more susceptible to listeriosis than the general public.

Hepatitis A can be transmitted by unsanitary food handling or by eating raw or undercooked shellfish harvested from contaminated waters.

One-cell parasites such as *Giardia lamblia*, found mainly in water, also infect HIV(+) individuals and people with AIDS.

The extent to which HIV(+) individuals are more at risk for each of these illnesses is unknown, but some scientists believe that any infection may hasten the progression from less severe HIV disease to AIDS.

Do's and Don'ts

Common-sense precautions in food selection and preparation can significantly lessen the hazard of infection from contaminated food. A cardinal rule is: Any raw animal-derived food must be considered to be contaminated with harmful microorganisms.

It is very dangerous for high-risk individuals to consume unpasteurized milk or raw or undercooked eggs, poultry, fish, shellfish, or meat.

The following food safety precautions are good advice for anyone, but they are especially important for people whose health is compromised, including people infected with HIV, cancer patients, people with diabetes, transplant recipients, infants, pregnant women, and the elderly.

1. Check displays, labels, and containers. Look for cleanliness at meat and seafood counters and salad bars. Proximity is important also. Cooked shrimp lying on the same bed of ice as raw fish could be contaminated.

2. Buy only Grade A or better eggs. Avoid eggs that are cracked or leaking.

3. Do not buy any foods whose "sell by" or "best used by" date has passed.

4. Read the label to see whether a food contains raw or undercooked animal-derived ingredients. Caesar salad dressing, for instance, traditionally uses raw eggs.

5. Buy only milk and cheeses labeled pasteurized. Cheese made of raw milk may be sold provided it has been aged for over 60 days. But AIDS patients should avoid this as well.

6. Keep groceries safe. Put raw seafood, poultry, and meat in plastic bags so drippings can not contaminate other foods in the shopping cart or bag.

7. Take groceries directly home and refrigerate cold foods. Hot foods from the deli should be eaten, kept hotter than 60° Celsius (140° Fahrenheit), or refrigerated right away. Leaving foods unrefrigerated for even a few hours fosters bacterial growth.

8. Store eggs in their original carton in the main section of the refrigerator. Do not put them in the egg section of the door because the temperature there is higher.

9. Be meticulously clean. Wash hands, utensils, counters, and cutting surfaces with hot soapy water between preparation of different foods, particularly after handling raw eggs,

meat, poultry, or fish. In other words, wash repeatedly during meal preparation to avoid cross-contamination.

10. Use glass cutting boards rather than wooden ones, which are difficult or impossible to clean adequately.

11. Be sure to disassemble and thoroughly wash the meat grinder and blender after grinding raw meat or poultry or blending eggs or vegetables.

12. Wash fresh fruits and vegetables with water, using a brush if appropriate.

13. Protect yourself with a plastic sealing bandage or plastic gloves if a hand has a cut or open sore, for wounds are easy entry points to the body for bacteria when handling raw meat, poultry, or fish.

14. Promptly refrigerate or cook foods, including vegetables, after you cut them up. Bacteria can grow at temperatures above 4° C (40° F) and below 60° C (140° F), so temperature is vital in keeping food safe.

   Using a thermometer, periodically check to make sure the temperature of your refrigerator is below 4° C (40° F) and the temperature of your freezer is no higher than minus 18° C (0° F).

15. Follow the recipe for seafood, but do not undercook it. Avoid lightly steamed mussels and snails, for instance. Fish should be flaky, not rubbery, when cut. Never eat oysters on the half shell, raw clams, sushi, or sashimi.

16. Cook eggs thoroughly until both the yolk and white are firm, not runny.

17. Reheat food or heat partially cooked foods all the way through to at least 74° C (165° F).

18. When cooking meat, follow the recipe's time and check temperature requirements, and check with a meat thermometer. Cook beef and lamb to at least 60° C (140° F), pork to 66° C (150° F), and poultry to 74° C (165° F). Use a meat thermometer to ensure complete cooking.

19. When using a microwave, observe the recipe's cooking time and directions about turning the dish.

20. When using a barbecue grill, precook meat and poultry. Refrigerate leftovers in covered containers to avoid cross-contamination.

21. Divide hot foods into small portions for quick cooling, and allow room for circulation around containers to prevent the refrigerator or freezer temperature from rising.

22. If food looks or smells suspicious, throw it out.

23. Take charge when dining out. As at home, do not eat uncooked animal-derived dishes, such as steak tartare, sushi, raw oysters, Hollandaise sauce, and homemade mayonnaise, eggnog, or ice cream. If you do not know what is in a particular dish, ask. Send back undercooked food—poultry, for instance — that is even slightly pink.

24. When ordering eggs, specify that scrambled eggs be dry and that fried eggs be well cooked on both sides. The runnier the yolk, the higher the risk.

25. Be extra careful during foreign travel. Check with your doctor before traveling to a foreign country. Do not buy food from street vendors. Avoid salads and raw vegetables, peel your own fruit, and only eat cooked food that is still hot. Drink only boiled or distilled or reverse osmosis bottled water and only use ice cubes made from boiled water.

26. A consumer or physician who believes an episode of diarrhea is related to a particular food or restaurant should tell the local health department or nearest FDA office. Such reporting can help others avoid the same illness.

Source: FDA Consumer, 1997.

Stop the Runs Before They Run You Down

by Nelson Vergel

Diarrhea is becoming one of the most common complaints of people taking protease inhibitors (Norvir and Viracept in particular). *In my experience with PoWeR clients, the number one reason for failure to gain lean body mass while on an anabolic program has been diarrhea.* This frustrating problem can really destroy a person's health and quality-of-life if not diagnosed and treated proactively. So, what can you do while your doctor is trying to find the cause of your diarrhea? There are many dietary considerations that you should know and that will make your life more bearable while you are experiencing this common problem.

According to Peter Anton, MD, a gastroenterologist and researcher at UCLA School of Medicine, 50 percent to 70 percent of HIV(+) individuals will, at some point, have recurrent diarrhea. Because diarrhea is usually caused by a variety of factors working together (infections, food problems, food allergies, drug side effects and/or other causes), aggressive diagnosis and treatment are crucial.

Bacterial Infections and Other Causes

It is very important to rule out infectious causes, so it is necessary to obtain analyses of three separate stool samples collected at approximately the same time on three successive days.

Cultures need to be ordered for parasites and their ova (eggs), usually abbreviated as O/P, and for typical bacterial pathogens (often called culture and sensitivity or C & S). Some labs that process samples from large immunocompromised populations automatically include investigations for *Cryptosporidia*, *Microsporidia*, *Isospora*, *Cyclospora* and *Giardia* (a common parasite). Other laboratories do not, so it is important for physicians to specifically request these tests.

Other causes of diarrhea are:

Bacterial Overgrowth — colonic bacteria sometimes travel to the relatively sterile small intestine, triggering diarrhea. A lactulose breath analyzer test can help diagnose this condition.

Functional Bowel Disease — not uncommon in HIV(+) people, this can cause rapid movement of liquids from the stomach through the intestines, resulting in diarrhea, along with gurgling, bloating, increased gas, feelings of urgency, and/or incomplete evacuation with bowel movements. The use of regular and slowly increasing doses of fiber (to help absorb the extra liquid and give more bulk to the stool) can help. Since this might be a factor, Dr. Anton recommends that one teaspoon of soluble fiber be consumed nightly, slowly increasing that amount weekly until the bowel frequency has slowed. A diet high in soluble fiber could also help.

HIV Effects — diarrhea may be secondary to the effects of HIV in the intestines. We often see diarrhea improve in people with AIDS when their previously high viral loads are reduced to undetectable levels.

For further diagnosis, Dr. Anton recommends an endoscopic evaluation, at least of the lower colon, be made. A more thorough evaluation to rule out infections would also include an upper endoscopy, something he strongly recommends if neither the above suggestions nor time result in improvement.

Recommended also is a Stool Analysis available with a prescription from your doctor from Great Smokies Lab (1-800-522-4762). Ask your doctor for the 3-day test that included parasites.

Dr. Lark Lands, one of America's top HIV nutrition experts, emphasizes that care must be taken in choosing foods and fluids, since the wrong kinds can make diarrhea worse. She includes these foods:

High-fat foods — Fat intolerance is a major cause of diarrhea; reducing fatty foods often results in substantial improvement.

Dairy products — Lactose intolerance is a frequent contributor to diarrhea and gas.

Hot, spicy foods — These can exacerbate diarrhea.

Acidic fruits — Oranges, grapefruits, and pineapples — and their juices. Limiting these can help reduce the stinging that makes diarrhea especially miserable.

Sugar — This sweetener will pull water from your system, the opposite of what you want if you have diarrhea.

Foods high in insoluble fiber — These increase the speed at which food travels through the intestines. Included are wheat bran, whole wheat products, popcorn, nuts, seeds, potato skins, corn, and a high intake of raw fruits and vegetables (especially their peels).

Helpful Foods

By contrast, foods that contain soluble fiber will often bring considerable improvement. They absorb water and expand, binding together the intestine's contents and slowing the passage of food. Included are fruits such as peeled apples or applesauce, peeled pears, apricots, peaches, plums, grapes, berries, melons, nectarines, prunes, and bananas, and such grain products as white rice, oatmeal, oat bran, and barley.

White rice and white bread, although lacking the higher levels of nutrients found in their whole-food counterparts, and thus not generally recommended for a healthful diet, may be temporarily useful as sources of calories that will not irritate the intestines. Mashed skinless potatoes are also non irritating calorie contributors.

Dr. Lands also recommends the BRAT diet for those with serious diarrhea who can find little that is tolerable. Every hour or so, eat small servings of banana (one soft one), boiled white rice (one-half cup), applesauce (one-half cup) and dry white toast (one slice). If plain white rice becomes boring, add flavor by cooling it with a beef or chicken bouillon cube and/or with flavorful herbs like bay leaf, dill weed, basil, or oregano. You could also add garlic powder or small amounts of soy or tomato sauce. Note that in some versions, the BRAT diet has an additional T, for tea. But since caffeine can exacerbate diarrhea, stick to a caffeine-free herbal variety.

No Flare-up Foods

Dr. James Scala, author of the book *Eating Right for a Bad Gut*, performed a survey among diarrhea sufferers. He tried to separate the foods into familiar groups that seem to make life better for folks with diarrhea. That is what led him to prepare a list of foods that most people could eat with no discomfort. He emphasizes that everyone can not eat all of them and some people need to eat almost any food in moderation. This listing shows that there are many foods to choose from. Foods are given by category with notes and pertinent facts about preparation.

Cereal: Oatmeal, Cream of Wheat, corn flakes, Bran Flakes, Malt O Meal, Special K, Product 19, and Cheerios. There is a clear avoidance of hard fiber (fiber matrix) wheat cereals.

Dairy Products: Lactaid milk, (many people use Lactaid milk sparingly), yogurt, aged cheese, cottage, and soft cheese.

Eggs: Some people have to avoid eggs because they can be highly allergenic.

Beef: Lean beef either as stew, roast, or steak, or ground and broiled or roasted. No frying.

Other Meat: Lean ham, carefully trimmed pork, and trimmed lamb. Emphasis is always put on lean and trimmed.

Fish. Fish is universally accepted. Fish that swim are called fin fish: They include tuna, swordfish, salmon, halibut, flounder and snapper. Preparation includes broiling, poaching, or baking. No fried fish!

Poultry: White meat of poultry with two provisions: the skin must be removed and the meat cannot be fried and breaded. Some people need to avoid dark poultry meat. Stewed, roasted, broiled, or grilled poultry is fine, but never fried.

Skin These Vegetables: Carrots, squash, tomatoes, cucumbers, celery and jicama. Remove skin and cook these vegetables until they are soft.

Vegetables with Skin: Broccoli, cauliflower, brussel sprouts, asparagus, all string beans, and peas. These vegetables must be cooked well by boiling. Steaming is acceptable for some folks, but the vegetables must be steamed until soft.

Beans: Some beans can simply be boiled: these include limas, navy beans, chickpeas, and lentils. Other beans, such as black, pinto, kidney, and red beans, must be cooked almost to a mush. Some people can eat canned baked beans. Be careful if gas is a problem (you may want to use Beano, a product found in stores that reduces flatulence).

Leafy Vegetables: Avoid leafy salads when there is diarrhea. Spinach is all right for most people when boiled or steamed well. Cabbage, if well cooked, is acceptable to a few people, but most insist they must avoid it at all costs (lots of gas!).

Potatoes: Potatoes are always eaten without the skin. Eat them baked, boiled, or mashed. Sweet potatoes and yams are fine if well cooked and peeled.

Fruits: It seems that most fruit is acceptable — if it is been peeled. Apples, pears, peaches (when peeled), avocados, bananas (if not green), apricots (if fully ripe and peeled), plums (if fully ripe and peeled), strawberries and kiwifruit, canned peaches, plums, pears, apples, oranges, and grapefruit. (Be careful to avoid the fibrous section in grapefruit.)

Grains: Boiled white and brown rice, pasta, egg noodles, and macaroni. Breads and rolls without seeds, including white, rye, wheat, five-grain, French, and Italian bread. Absolutely no seeds of any type: sesame, poppy, etc.

Processed Foods: Try to avoid processed foods, but there are some that can be used: canned fruit, canned applesauce, and baked beans for some people. Pretzels, bagels, and some mildly sweet cookies may be fine. No chocolate chips!

Beverages: Most people can use fruit juices, and vegetable juices, such as tomato and V-8 juice. Specific fruit juices were orange, cranberry, and apple. Some people are allergic to apple juice and citrus juices, though. Tea, caffeine-free tea, iced and hot, not strong; caffeine-free cola and other carbonated beverages, mineral water and distilled water are also okay.

Supplements

While your doctor is looking for the cause of your diarrhea, there are many things you can supplement your diet to minimize it. Some of the following have been discussed in other sections of the book. They include:

L-glutamine: This amino acid acts like a fertilizer for your intestinal walls, which are eroded by frequent bowel movements. We have seen good results in our clients who have taken 30-50 grams a day in divided doses. (One heaping tablespoon is 12 grams.)

Digestive enzymes: These can help digest proteins, carbohydrates, and fats, which tend to pass through the digestive track quickly when you are having diarrhea. Good products are made by Jarrow, Enzymatic Therapy and Absorbaid.

Undenatured, immunoglobulin-rich, whey protein: Optimune whey protein has been developed to actively help fight pathogens in your gut to reduce or eliminate diarrhea. Doses of 20 to 60 grams per day are recommended. Optimune will cause some people who are allergic to dairy to have more diarrhea.

Stanozolol (Winstrol): Oral anabolic steroid that seems to have more anticatabolic effects than some other steroids, which seems to help minimize weight loss resulting from diarrhea. Available by prescription, 4 mg three times per day for men, or 2 mg three times per day for women seems to be effective.

Acidophilus: Friendly bacteria used to increase good flora in your gut that compete with bugs that can cause diarrhea. Take 20 minutes before every meal. Keep refrigerated.

Hydrating drinks: Drink lots of distilled, reverse osmosis or preboiled water, or soups, to keep yourself hydrated during bouts of diarrhea. Dehydration will zap your energy, and will cause you to lose electrolytes.

Psyllium: Provides bulk fiber and absorbs water. Contained in Metamucyl. Do not take two hours before or one hour after taking medications or vitamins because psyllium can bind them and stop their absorption.

Electrolyte supplements: Replacing electrolytes can be critical to recovery. Scientifically designed electrolyte formulas are SuperNutrition Super C (from health food stores and buyers' clubs), and Pedialyte (from drug stores). Super C tastes like lemon. Pedialyte does not taste good.

Growth hormone: As mentioned before, growth hormone may help reduce diarrhea and improve the health of the intestines, but again, to reduce the potential for side effects, find the lowest replacement dose that gets the desired effect. Usually this will be between 0.5 mg and 3 mg per day.

As you can tell, there is a lot you can do to minimize the destructive effects of diarrhea, even with an undiagnosed cause. Watching what you eat, taking a few very good supplements, and drinking lots of caffeine-free fluids will help you stop the runs before they run you down.

Getting Started: What to Do Before You Start the PoWeR Program

by Nelson Vergel

1. Read this book carefully. Learn about anabolic steroids, nutrition, supplements, and the exercise aspects of the program.

2. Get a baseline bioelectrical impedance analysis (BIA) done to determine your body composition. Get it done again every three months after that. Call the largest HIV/AIDS organization near you and ask them for a referral to a nutritionist or dietitian. They usually have access to BIA and nutritional software that can give you some guidelines. Call RJL at 1-800-790-0205 and ask them who does BIA in your city. (RJL has this information as they sell the machine to doctors, institutions, and dietitians)

3. Call one of the buyer's clubs to order a high-potency vitamin product (the best buy and the best formulas are the SuperNutrition Opti-Pack and the SuperNutrition Super Blend). If you need extra protein, get a protein powder supplement.

4. For those of you who wish to participate in the use of anabolic steroids, you are encouraged to enroll your own physician. Present the PoWeR *Anabolic Hormone Guidelines* to your physician. If your physician will not prescribe steroids, be aware that there are a number of physicians that will prescribe anabolic steroids for wasting due to HIV disease. Call the Houston Buyers' Club at 1-800-350-2392 for a referral to a doctor in your area.

5. Get a testosterone and a free testosterone test, and a DHEA-S test.

6. The prescription for the PoWeR cycle (testosterone + nandrolone) should include nandrolone decanoate (Deca-Durabolin — 12 vials of 200 mg/ml, as directed), and testosterone enanthate or cypionate (Depo-Testosterone), 10 cc's, 200 mg/ml, 2 bottles, as directed). To inject this, get at least 50 syringes (23-gauge, 1 inch). Also get vitamin B-12 (30 cc's, 1000 mcg/ml, 1 vial, 1 or more 1 cc shots per week). To inject this, get at least 24 ultra-fine insulin syringes.

Ask your doctor or their nurse to teach you to give yourself the injections, or have them teach your lover or a close friend how to do it correctly. The entire PoWeR cycle for three months can cost under $500 if you have to pay for it.

7. If your testosterone and free testosterone tested as being normal before you started using steroids, which may mean that you do not need to be on permanent testosterone replacement,

you will also need to get the materials that can help restart your natural testosterone production that are used in the refractory protocol on page 75. These include human chorionic gonadotropin (HCG) — 2 vials of 10,000 USP, injected with ultra-fine syringes; Clomid — 56 of the 50 mg tablets, and Arimidex—56 of the 1 mg tablets. Note that this adds more cost to the cycle.

8. Join a gym, if you do not already have a membership. Get a workout partner or if you have the money, get a personal trainer. Follow the exercise recommendations described in the PoWeR book, and learn all you can about proper weight-training. The YMCA has a scholarship or reduced rate program for people who have a low income or are on disability.

Weight-Lifting for Maximum Muscle Gains

A Simple, But Effective Method

by Michael Mooney

In this section I present a simple yet effective weight-lifting program. You can modify this program after you have gotten your initial muscle gains. You will then be familiar with the new body you are building and how it responds to weight-training whether you are using steroids or not. It is best to start this program slowly, then gradually increase intensity over several weeks or months. At the end of this section, I provide details on how to perform the individual exercises correctly so that you get the best results safely. I want to emphasize that this program is suggested as a starting point. After you are familiar with your body, and the exercises, you are invited to experiment with different weight-lifting methods and learn how to modify your program to keep your body growing while you learn to shape your muscles. Elite coaches vary their athletes' programs constantly. Once you get an exercise foundation, you should too.

Beginning Exercise At Home

For people who are very fragile and in the beginning stages of recovering functional strength, I recommend a copy of the video titled *Exercises for People with HIV By People With HIV*. This video was created specifically for HIV(+) people. It demonstrates a simple, well-balanced exercise program for beginners that you can do at home. It incorporates mind/body movements from chi kung and weight-lifting movements that you can do with hand weights or light dumbbells. People who have lost the feeling of fundamental strength that most of us take for granted will find this video to be the perfect motivational tool to help you start rebuilding your body. To obtain this video, call 1 (404) 876-5192.

Safety First!

Always remember, *safety first*. If something you do in an exercise hurts, stop! Ask for help to figure out what you are doing wrong. Maybe it is just improper form. *If you hurt yourself you will hinder your progress because you will not be about to work out!*

Commit Yourself

First priority is to join a gym if you can afford it. If you spend money on a membership, you will be more likely to stay with it, and consistency is the key to success in any exercise program. Also, try to find someone who is enthusiastic to train with, or get a personal trainer (if you can afford the additional expense). It is easier to stay motivated when you train with someone else who has a vital interest in your mutual success. It is also safer to have someone spot you when you lift heavy weights.

Train Smart — Do Not Overtrain!

Overtraining is probably the most ignored limiting factor. And it is especially important to avoid overtraining because HIV disease tends to create the same kind of catabolic effect on muscle tissue that overtraining does. Overtraining, which is the same thing as overstressing, can lower immune response and cause the loss of muscle tissue.

Often times people think that they are not training hard enough, so they increase the number of exercise routines that they perform in the belief that they just need more stimulus! This is one of the biggest errors a person can make — more is *not* necessarily better! It seems paradoxical that you could work out less and grow more, but this is very often the case.

Any amount of exercise beyond that which is the amount of stimulus necessary to induce optimal muscle growth can be called overtraining. Let me repeat that: exercising more than what the body requires to stimulate it maximally to grow is overtraining. Keep your program simple, work out hard, do just the right amount of exercise to stimulate growth, and you will succeed.

Proper Stimulus

In order to build muscle, the body has to receive a stimulus — a reason — to grow bigger, to achieve what is called hypertrophy. It is really very simple: the body only does what it needs to do — what it is required to do. It is not going to suddenly expand its muscle mass because it anticipates needing more muscles. But if it is challenged to move weight, it will respond by growing. Another way to look at it is if you take any bodybuilder and put him in bed for weeks at a time, he will begin to lose muscle mass — because the body will sense it does not need the extra muscle anymore. You need to deliver the stimulus to provoke muscular growth in the body — and that is what lifting weights does.

Aerobics Versus Weight-Lifting

Exercise as weight-training can improve lean body mass for HIV(+) people without the use of anabolic steroids.[1-3] And, while aerobic exercise also can improve overall health if not carried to excess (overtraining), it does not appreciably improve lean body mass, and it can drain some of the limited energy that the body would use to grow muscle. So when a person is wasting or recovering from illness, aerobics should be eliminated entirely, *as it can cause a serious decrease in muscle growth rate and often times a loss of muscle for the person who is metabolically challenged.*

Once you have stable, healthy lean body mass, for fat loss I suggest 20 to 30 minutes of aerobics, three times per week, first thing in the morning before eating breakfast. Doing aerobics with an empty stomach increases the fat loss tremendously as the body has used up much of its reserve fuels in sleep, so it will burn fat more efficiently. But if you eat carbohydrates before you do aerobics you will burn the carbohydrates when they get into your bloodstream rather than your own fat. I also recommend doing aerobics on alternate days to weight-lifting, as this keeps you from overstressing your metabolism (overtraining).

Set Goals

Create a roadmap that will keep you on track and moving forward by setting reasonable goals for the total increase in muscle mass and body weight you are striving for. Once you get familiar with the amount you are capable of lifting when you start, set goals for the amount of weight you want to be able to lift.

A Workout Journal

Logging your workouts in a journal will help you work out better. The best reason to keep track of your workouts is so that you can see what you are accomplishing. The journal also helps you stay focused so that you can zero in on your goals, that is, you program your mind when you look at black and white. You will also be able to see whether you are gaining at a reasonable rate or you see whether you are overtraining; if so you will not be gaining in strength, and this will add up to not gaining in muscle size. So keep a journal of your workouts: write down the weight poundage you lift and the amount of repetitions (reps) you lift for each exercise. Then, when you go in to train again the next week, you know what numbers you are trying to better. If you find out that you are weaker than you were the time before, and everything else is in line, you may be training too often. One ready-made, well-designed journal that can help you track your workouts is *The Muscle and Might Training Tracker* by Stuart McRobert, available for $23.95 by credit card at www.hardgainer.com or by calling 1-509-234-0362 or by mailing to CS Publishing, P.O. Box 1002, Connell, WA 99326.

Starters: Once-A-Week Training

This section is for those who have only recently recovered from illness, or are just getting into weight-lifting for the first time. For the first few weeks, until your stamina is up, do only one workout per week. The workout described below is a whole-body workout program. For more descriptions of various exercises get a book like *The Gold's Gym Training Encyclopedia* that details proper form for the full spectrum of resistance exercises, by calling 1-800-496-8734.

Warm-up set (w) weight refers to a set where you use a weight that is about 50 to 60 percent of the heavy weight set that you use. Heavy (h) indicates a weight that you are only capable of lifting 6 to 12 times before you experience momentary muscular failure.

1. Barbell flat bench press — 2 w and 1 h set
2. Curl-grip pulldowns — 2 w and 1 h set
3. Squat or seated leg press — 2 w and 1 h set
   Squats are a best exercise, but some people have to substitute the leg press because their back or knees will not tolerate squats.

Warm-up sets employ a poundage that you know you can *easily* handle for 12 repetitions (reps). Rest for about one minute between sets or longer — until you feel like you have enough energy to go again. Two warm-up sets should be enough to warm all the joints involved without tiring you too much. Then do the heavy set. You want to lift the weight until you can not lift it again. This is called momentary muscular failure.

Your Personal Best

After you get used to training, it is important to challenge yourself to the best of your own ability and do enough repetitions to get to momentary muscular failure so that you trigger your muscles to grow. Your level of intensity in the beginning will not be as great as it can be later, after you have been at it for a while. Give yourself time, and allow yourself to grow slowly, but do work to the best of your own ability. You do not have to go to the point of total failure, where you can not even hold the weight in place to gain muscle. In fact, this is a form of overtraining, and is a technique to be used only on very rare occasions.

Do this workout on a day when you feel relatively good. After doing the exercises, you may feel tired and depleted. You should consume a low-fat carbohydrate/protein drink after the workout to replenish glycogen (muscle sugar) and amino acid stores — you will grow much better if you do. A good drink mix is OSMO Regeneration (contains no aspartame), which is sold at health food stores and buyers' clubs like the Houston Buyer's Club, 1-800-350-2392.

If you find that you feel exhausted during your beginning efforts, pace yourself more carefully and make sure your nutrition and rest are good. You should be getting balanced nutrition (like food!) three to six times a day and be sure to get plenty of rest and recovery. Protein drinks can fill in between meals. (e.g. three meals with two or three drinks per day.) Continue with once-a-week workouts until you find that you feel good enough to workout on a second, non-consecutive day of the week. Then do this same workout twice a week. When you feel good enough to workout three days a week, it is time to start splitting the exercise routine up to work on one group of body parts per day. You will also be starting to train your heavy sets with more intensity, and you will see an acceleration of the muscular gains. After you have been training for a while, say three to six months, begin to experiment with different training programs, combinations of exercises, and techniques. There are many different valid ways to train, and each has something to offer. A interesting book on sophisticated training approaches is *The Poliquin Principles* by Charles Poliquin. To order it call 1-707-257-2348. Another book with an entirely different, more fundamental approach to training is *Beyond Brawn* by Stuart McRobert, ordered by credit card at www.hardgainer.com, or by calling 1-509-234-0362, or by mailing to CS Publishing, P.O. Box 1002, Connell, WA 99326.

THE 3-DAY SPLIT

On several of these exercises I give you an alternate exercise to use for variety. In the beginning, you should probably stick with one specific exercise for a given body part for a period of four to eight weeks, then use an alternate. Once you become familiar with weight-lifting and correct technique, you will want to try some of the other many different variations and perhaps begin to periodize your training and use more advanced techniques.

Day 1: Chest, Shoulders, Triceps
    Barbell flat bench press — 2 w and 1 h set
    (Alternate: incline bench press)
    Cable side deltoid raise (laterals) — 2 w and 1 h set
    Cable rear deltoid raises — 2 w and 1 h set
    Triceps pushdowns — 2 w and 1 h set
    (Alternate: Close-grip bench press)
    Note: Rest one or more days.

Day 2: Back, Biceps, Abdominals
    Seated close-grip pulldowns to the stomach — 2 w and 1 h set
    Barbell biceps curl — 2 w and 1 h set
    (Alternate: preacher bench barbell curls)
    Crunches — 3 sets of 10-20 reps
    Note: Rest one or more days.

Day 3: Quadriceps, Hamstrings, and Calves (Legs)
    Squat — 2 w and 1 h set
    (Alternate: Seated leg press)
    Again, the squat is the better overall exercise, but some people cannot do it because of back or knee problems.
    Lying leg curls — 2 w and 1 h set
    Standing calf raises — 2 w and 1 h set
    Note: Legs are the most demanding body part, so rest two or more days.

Control The Weight

Studies show that the negative, or return part of the movement is critical to optimal muscle growth, so do not let the weight fall quickly after lifting it. Exert deliberate control over the negative part of the movement, keeping tension on your muscles through the full range of the movement, and do not rush it.

Making Progress

When you can lift a weight for twelve reps, raise the weight 5 to 10 pounds so that you can only lift about six reps. Then try to increase the number of reps you can lift each time you work out to arrive at twelve reps again, and repeat the progression so that you keep increasing the weight you lift. As you grow stronger, you will grow bigger muscles. You will probably be pretty sore during your early recovery days. For best recovery and growth let yourself heal so that the soreness goes away, even if this means you leave several days between workouts.

During one high-intensity training period several years ago I learned by studying my workout records that if I wanted to put on weight most quickly, I needed a minimum of eight-days of rest before I worked the same body part. This meant that for the type of training I was doing I worked a body part every nine days. If you do not allow enough recovery days between workouts, your progress will be slower. When you log your workouts you can see if you are progressing. If you are not making progress pretty much every workout, try giving yourself another day to recover and see if you do not get stronger at each workout. A very thin, ectomorphic guy I once counseled needed 14 days between workouts to grow optimally!

Keep in mind that the goal is to gain strength and lean body mass. Usually strength precedes size, so you get stronger and then notice that you are getting bigger.

Weight-Lifting Exercises

Flat Bench Barbell Press

This exercise primarily works the pectorals or chest. The anterior deltoids and triceps are also involved. Grip should be a little wider than shoulder width.

Steps: Lie down on your back on a flat bench, with your feet flat on floor.
Put your hands on bar slightly wider than your shoulders.
Pick up the bar by extending your arms. Lift the weight straight up over your chest for a count of one.
Squeeze your chest at the top, hold 1-2 seconds.
Slowly lower the bar (over 2 seconds), by allowing your elbows to flare out away from your body until your upper arm is parallel to floor. Keep your elbows up toward your shoulders rather than letting them flex down toward stomach.
Repeat.

Alternate: Incline Bench Press

This exercise is basically the same as the flat bench press, but tends to work the upper chest and front of the shoulders a little more.

Cable Side Deltoid Raises (Laterals)

This exercise builds the side deltoid cap, the muscle that gives the wide look — think of cannonball delts. This is not an easy exercise to get at first, but once you learn it you will find it to be a best exercise for shoulders, and it *is* better than lateral raises with dumbbells.

Steps: With a single handle that is attached to a low cable pulley, and leaning slightly forward (with your left side nearest the cable frame), raise the cable from a position to the side of your stomach up and to the outside of your right shoulder. Do this as if you were swinging a back fist so that you would hit someone behind you with the back of your hand. Be sure to swing the cable in an arc out in front of your body with your arm almost straight, with a slight flex in the elbow rather than letting it stay low as it comes around. Feel yourself resisting the pull of gravity as you move through this arc.
The position you end at should be about shoulder height out to your right. Hold 1-2 seconds.
Control the negative movement as you let the cable pull your arm in an arc back down to the left side of your stomach to the starting position (over 2 seconds).
Repeat.
Repeat the entire sequence for the other side, but reverse your position.

Cable Rear Deltoid Raises

This exercise builds your rear deltoid so that you have a deep and wide look. You may see people who seem to have big shoulder caps, but when they turn sideways they disappear. The rear delt completes the shoulders and makes them look much more powerful. Many people miss this.

Steps: With a single handle that is attached to a low cable pulley, and bent over at the waist so that your torso is horizontal, with your left side nearest the cable frame, pull the cable from a position under your body to the left of your left shoulder in an arc up to the outside of your right shoulder. Keep your arm straight or only slightly bent throughout the movement. Avoid flexing your tricep during the movement.

Your hand should end at a high position — on the same plane as your head, not down by your stomach. Hold 1-2 seconds.

Control the negative movement as you let the cable pull your arm in an arc back down to the side of your left shoulder at the starting position (over 2 seconds).

Repeat.

Repeat the entire sequence for the other side, but reverse your position.

Triceps Cable Pushdown

This exercise effectively works the triceps as long as you keep the elbows close to the body during the movement. Do this exercise with a bent bar that has a bend in the middle so that it is shaped like a slight V.

Steps: Stand with your feet hip width apart, bend knees slightly, and put your back to the pad at the overhead pulley machine.

Grasp the V-handle bar with overhand grip, palms facing downward.

Pull your shoulder blades back, lift chest, and tighten abdominals.

By contracting your triceps, straighten your arms, aggressively pushing bar down toward floor.

Stop when your arms are fully extended.

Squeeze your triceps, hold 1-2 seconds.

Without moving upper arms, return to starting position (over 2 seconds).

Repeat.

Close-grip Bench Press

This exercise works the triceps with some involvement of the shoulders and chest. Performed somewhat like the standard bench press, only with a closer grip.

Steps: With a grip approximately 14 inches apart, no closer, lower the barbell from over your chest keeping your arms close to your body. The bar should end at a spot just below

your pecs, before driving it back up to a lockout position; this keeps the tension on the inner chest and triceps, which is right where you want it.

Squeeze your triceps. Hold 1-2 seconds.

Return to the starting position (over 2 seconds).

Repeat.

Seated Close-grip Overhead Cable Pulldowns

If done properly, this exercise works the entire back (lats).

Steps: Sit on bench with feet flat on floor, abdominals tight.

Grasp overhead pulley bar with hands about eight inches apart with palms facing you.

From the fully stretched overhead position, pull the bar down to your stomach by bringing your elbows to your sides as you lean back slightly. Be sure to keep your back arched and firm with your shoulders back.

Squeeze your lats in the bottom position. Hold 1-2 seconds.

Keeping your back firm, slowly (over 2 seconds) let the bar go up until you are in the fully stretched overhead starting position.

Repeat.

Standing Barbell Curls

This exercise primarily works the biceps. The EZ curl bar is best for this but a straight bar can be used.

Steps: Grasp barbell slightly wider than shoulder width, palms facing forward. Pull shoulders back, lift chest. Arms should be fully straightened down at your sides.

Stand with feet hip width apart, bend knees slightly, tighten abdominals.

By contracting biceps, slowly move barbell in an arc out from the front of the body until the barbell is up to your chest. The hard part is to keep elbows at your sides (stationary) throughout the movement. That is why it is easier to do curls using a bench.

Squeeze your biceps at the top, hold 1-2 seconds, keeping your elbows stationary.
Slowly return to starting position (over 2 seconds).
Repeat.

Preacher Curl

This exercise works the biceps. All assisting muscles are removed from any involvement in this lift, so this isolates the biceps very well. The EZ curl bar is best for this, but a straight bar can be used. Bring the weight all the way to the bottom fully stretched position for full development of the biceps. For any exercise to fully develop a given muscle, it must to through the full range of motion. If you do not go all the way to the bottom, the lower part of the biceps will not grow as well. Control the weight and do not jerk on the way to the bottom as this can cause injury.

Steps: From the seated position of the preacher bench, grasp the EZ curl barbell at the outside grip position, palms facing forward.
By contracting biceps, lift the barbell up to the topmost position.
Squeeze your biceps at top and hold 1-2 seconds.
Slowly return to the bottom at the starting position (over 2 seconds). Be sure to go all the way down smoothly.
Repeat.

Abdominal Crunches on Mat

Primarily works the abdominals.

Steps: Lie flat on your back.
Bend knees 90 degrees.
Press lower back into floor.
Tighten abdominals.
Slowly curl upper body towards pelvis, leaving lower back on mat.
When your head is highest off the mat, squeeze your abdominals. Hold 1-2 seconds.
Slowly curl your upper body back to the starting position.
Repeat.
Note: concentrate on squeezing your abdominals throughout the movement.

Barbell Squats

This most taxing of all exercises primarily works the quadriceps (thigh), but it also involves the gluteals (buttocks), and hamstrings. This is the exercise that can best reverse AZT butt! It is a difficult exercise that not everyone can perform. Tall lanky people often have trouble doing squats. I recommend the assistance of a competent spotter.

Steps: Stand up straight with your feet hip width apart. Face straight bar on squat rack.
Place midpoint of bar across your trapezius muscle (back of neck/shoulder).
Place your hands wider than shoulder width to balance the bar, your palms facing forward to grasp the bar.
Place your feet hip width apart, facing forward with your knees lined up over your toes.
Pull your shoulder blades back, arch your back, chest up, and tighten your abdominals.
By bending your knees, smoothly descend to a position where your upper legs are parallel to the floor (about 2 seconds). Be sure to look straight ahead, not down, keep your chest lifted, and maintain a slight arch in your lower back.
Contract your quadriceps, and straighten your legs to lift you up to the starting position, as though you are trying to push your feet through the floor (over 1 second).
Repeat.

Squats are a difficult exercise to learn to do properly and a short description does not really do it justice. One good book to read to learn to squat properly is "The Insider's Tell-All Handbook on Weight-Training Technique," by Stuart McRobert. You can get it by credit card at www.hardgainer.com or by calling 1-509-234-0362 or by mailing to CS Publishing, P.O. Box 1002, Connell, WA 99326. Another one is "Super Squats," by Randall Strossen, Ph.D., ordered by calling 1-800-447-0008, ext. 1.

Seated Leg Press

This exercise primarily works the quadriceps (or thigh), but it also involves the hamstrings and gluteals. This puts less strain on the back than squats.

Steps: Sit on the machine with your lower back and shoulders against the pad.

Place your feet hip width apart on the platform. Contract your quadriceps and straighten your knees to lift the weight to starting position.

Pull your shoulders back, tighten your abdominals. Lower the weight by smoothly bending your knees as your legs come down toward your chest (2 seconds).

Stop just before your knees touch your chest.

Contract your quadriceps and straighten your knees to lift the weight.

For maximal effect do not straighten your legs fully, but shop short of lockout and hold for 1-2 seconds. This stresses the quads more.

Repeat.

Lying Leg Curl Machine

This exercise works the hamstrings (leg biceps).

Steps: Lie on the leg curl machine, placing the back of your ankles under the pad.

Press your abdominals tightly down onto the machine.

By contracting hamstrings, slowly bring heels toward buttocks. Stop when you are unable to bring your heels any closer without moving your abdominals. Keep your hips in contact with the machine at all times.

Squeeze hamstrings. Hold 1-2 seconds.

Slowly return to the starting position (2 seconds).

Repeat.

Standing Calf Machine

This exercise works both heads of the calf.

Steps: Stand with your toes on the platform, your heels off the platform, and your knees slightly bent, with the pad on your shoulders.

Pull your shoulders back, tighten your abdominals.

By contracting your calves, rise up on your toes (1 second).

Stop when you are as high as you can get on your tiptoes. Squeeze your calves and hold 1-2 seconds

Slowly return to the starting position (2 seconds).

Repeat.

RECOMMENDED READING

Below we list some good basic references so that you may gather all the information you need to make informed decisions about the use of our guidelines. *We do not agree with everything in these publications*, and our concepts may differ considerably with some concepts they contain. However, they all have some merit. If you have questions about anything in these books that is related to our guidelines, you may call the PoWeR question and answer hotline at (310) 360-0654.

AIDS — Immune System

1. *Healing HIV*, by Jon Kaiser, M.D. Health First Press. Mill Valley, California. Jon's second book shows tremendous evolution in his approach. His wellness-based integrated HIV medical model is designed to build health and strength in the body so that you either do not need to use AIDS drugs or you respond better to lower doses of drugs. Dr. Kaiser believes that you will also have less potential to become resistant to the drugs that are needed. His ideas about addressing hormonal and nutritional deficiencies and improving digestive health should be studied by HIV(+) people and their doctors.

2. *Dr. Jon Kaiser's Newsletter.* Send a card requesting a free subscription to Health First Press, 775 East Blithedale, Suite 367, Mill Valley, CA 94941.

3. *Surviving with AIDS*, by Wayne Callaway, M.D. Little, Brown and Company, Boston.

4. *The Guide to Living with HIV Infection*, by John Bartlett, M.D. The Johns Hopkins University Press. 701 West 40th Street, Baltimore, MD 21211.

5. *The AIDS Fighters*, by Ian Brightope, M.D. Keats Publishing, Inc., New Canaan, CT 06840.

6. *How Your Immune System Works*, by Jeff Baggish, M.D. Ziff-Davis Press, 5903 Christie Avenue, Emeryville, CA 94608. This insightful doctor/author also illustrated this book. It is understandable to everyone.

7. *500 Tips for Coping with Chronic Illness*, by Pamela Jacobs, M.A. Robert Read Publishers, 750 La Playa, Suite 647, San Francisco, CA 94121.

8. *AIDS Treatment News* The best single, quick periodical devoted to AIDS research. 1 (415) 255-0588.

9. *Cooking For Life*, A Guide To Nutrition and Food Safety for the HIV-Positive Community, by Robert H. Lehmann. Dell Publishing. Available at most large book stores.

Nutrition

1. *Mastering The Zone*, by Barry Sears, Ph.D. Harper Collins Publishers, Inc., 10 East 53rd, Street, New York, NY 10022. Learn the prin-

ciples but avoid the dogma. Numerous people have told us how they have reduced their lipodystrophy symptoms and/or lowered their cholesterol using the "zone" approach to eating. To build muscle, eat more calories than he recommends, though.

2. *The Fat Burning Diet*, by Jay Robb. Jay Robb Enterprises, Box 711533, Santee, CA 92072-1533. Call 1 (800) 862-8763 to order. Similar principles as the Zone diet, but not as rigid. Could also be called *Fat-Burning, Muscle Building Diet,* as the information in this book can also apply to building muscle if you get enough calories.

4. *Optimum Sports Nutrition*, by Michael Colgan, Ph.D. Advanced Research Press, 2120 Smithtown Avenue, Ronkonkoma, NY 11779. Dr. Colgan is one of the most accurate and innovative general health and sports nutrition writers, and his books all have something interesting to offer. We disagree with much of what he says about steroids, though.

5. *Nutrients as Ergogenic Aids for Sports and Exercise*, by Luke Bucci, Ph.D. CRC Press, Inc. 2000 Corporate Boulevard, N.W. Boca Raton, FL 33431.

6. *Fats that Heal, Fats that Kill*, by Udo Erasmus. Alive Books, 7436 Fraser Park Drive, Burnaby BC Canada V5J 5B9. This book details how essential fatty acids are critical for optimal health.

7. Healing Nutrients, by Patrick Quillin, Ph.D. Random House Publishers, New York, NY.

8. *Flax Oil as a True Aid Against Arthritis, Heart Infarction, Cancer, and Other Diseases*, by Dr. Joanna Budwig. Apple Publishing Company Ltd. 220 East 50th Avenue, Vancouver, British Columbia, Canada V5X 1X9.

9. *Prescription for Nutritional Healing*, by James Balch, M.D. Avery Publishing Group, Inc., Garden City Park, New York.

10. *Nutrition Almanac*, by Lavon J. Dunne. McGraw-Hill Publishing Company, New York, NY.

11. *Sports Supplement Review,* by Bill Phillips. The fact that this book is a very good sales tool for Bill's EAS bodybuilding supplements does not change the fact that he and his staff have produced an insightful guide to bodybuilding supplements that really is the best of its kind. 1 (800) 297-9776.

12. *The Green Pharmacy*, by James Duke, Ph.D. Prevention Books. Available at any book store. Botanist and former head of the U.S. Department of Agriculture James Duke promotes natural healing with foods and herbs.

13. *Alternative Medicine*. This is one of the best magazines to subscribe to if you are interested in nutrition and alternative or complementary medicine. 1 (360) 385-6021.

14. *Townsend Letter for Doctors and Patients*. Alternative (nutritional) medicine's oldest journal. 1 (360) 385-6021.

15. *Clinical Pearls News*. CP reviews 5,000 journals and gives a brief synopsis of interesting nutrition studies. Highly recommended. 1 (916) 483-1431.

Anabolic Steroids

1. *Beyond Anabolic Steroids*, by Dr. Mauro Di Pasquale. M.G.D. Press, 23 Main Street, Warkworth, Ontario K0K 3K0. Dr. Di Pasquale is one of the most accurate researchers there is, and each of his books is worthwhile reading.

2. *Anabolic Steroid Side Effects*, by Dr. Mauro Di Pasquale. M.G.D. Press, 23 Main Street, Warkworth, Ontario K0K 3K0.

3. Anabolic-Androgenic Steroids, by Charles Kochakian, Ph.D., Springer-Verlag, Berlin 1976, ISBN 3-540-07710-3. This out-of-print book, edited by the father of anabolic steroids, Dr. Charles Kochakian, starts with the details of Dr. Kochakian's early discoveries in 1935 and provides a solid foundation to understand the metabolism of testosterone and its analogs. Of the numerous academic books on anabolic steroids that could be recommended, including books by Kruskemper, Vida, and others, this is perhaps the best book to read.

4. *Anabolic Reference Guide*, by Bill Philips. Mile High Publishing. P.O. Box 277, Golden, Colorado 80402. A comprehensive underground guide to the different anabolic steroids. Does not provide medical information, though.

5. *The Underground Steroid Handbook*, by Dan Duchaine. This is the most popular underground steroid book of all time because of Dan's irreverence, and the way he tells it like it is.

Note: All the currently available underground steroid books contain significant scientific errors. Most of the information they contain is based on anecdotal information rather than medical journal studies, so use them as general guides only.

Weight-Training

1. *The Poliquin Principles*, by Charles Poliquin. Charles Poliquin is an expert physical training coach to elite athletes and Olympic champions. His approach is extremely creative (and humorous). This is a good source of sophisticated weight-training techniques. 1 (707) 257-2348.

2. *Heavy-Duty*, by Mike Mentzer. Mike's controversial approach can work very well in its context. Is it the only correct method as Mentzer says it is? Michael Mooney trained with Mentzer for 10 weeks in 1994 and got amazing increases in strength. Elite training coaches like Charles Poliquin and Dragomir Cioroslan credibly contend that building and fine-tuning a physique for strength, aesthetics or competition requires a more varied approach. While we agree with them, you can learn something valuable from Mentzer's approach — and it is simple. Call 1 (310) 827-7661.

3. *Muscle Meets Magnet*, by Per Tesch, Ph.D. This book uses magnetic resonance imaging (MRI) to show you how certain exercises affect specific muscles. This will help you understand correct training form and how you can target your muscles to shape them for best balance. 1 (800) 447-0008, ext.1.

4. *The Gold's Gym Training Encyclopedia.* This book has basic details on proper form and technique, and tells you which exercises affect which muscles giving you a full spectrum of resistance exercises. 1(800) 496-8734.

5. *Getting Stronger* by Bill Pearl. Great pictures, easy to read, great price. 1(800) 496-8734 or www.amazon.com.

Our Newsletter - MEDIBOLICS

Our medical anabolic research newsletter provides updates to this book and new research information covering all aspects of gaining lean muscle mass for wasting caused by AIDS and other diseases. Topics we cover include anabolic drugs, nutrition, dietary supplements, weight-training, and political issues related to health-care. Updated versions of articles taken from different issues of Medibolics are reprinted in this book.

See selected articles from Medibolics on the internet at **http://www.medibolics.com**.

Contents:

- Party drug Special K (ketamine) — Does it lower natural killer cells?
- What steroid dose is too high?
- A doctor answers questions about her patients' steroid experiences
- Glutamine supplementation and the immune system

Volume 2, Number 1 (Issue 5)
- Oxandrin — higher doses needed
- Is Winstrol better than Oxandrin?
- The First International Wasting Conference
- PoWeR wellness center to open
- DHEA and androstenedione
- Protease inhibitors cause fat gain
- Megace w/testosterone still causes fat gain
- Spray vitamins
- Testosterone injections — How often?
- Medical-grade whey protein
- President Clinton declares war on doctors
- Testosterone before transfusions
- Steroids, the liver, and supplements
- Nelson Vergel detained at U.S. Customs

Volume 2, Number 2 (Issue 6)
- Why protease inhibitors might cause potbelly
- Androstenedione lab tests
- Testosterone may reduce loss of T cells
- The return of the guerilla steroid — Anadrol
- Study — glutamine promotes weight gain
- The trouble with vanadyl
- Testosterone before other steroids
- Muscle Media changes

Volume 2, Number 3 (Issue 7)
- Appetite Stimulants — Marinol, Megace and medicinal marijuana
- Cost and weight gain comparison of growth hormone and steroids
- Growth hormone kickbacks
- Lipodystrophy, cardiovascular disease, growth hormone, and anabolic steroids
- More on Anadrol-50
- Viagra with testosterone
- Do oral GH boosters (ProhGH and Regenesis) work?
- Women's estrogen replacement therapy increases mortality
- Heard in Geneva: Oxandrin causes liver toxicity
- Steroids may decrease protease inhibitor belly

To Subscribe

The cost for a subscription is $20 for four issues, payable in cash, check or money order. Back issues are $5 each. The U.S. and foreign subscriber rates are the same. Send to: Medibolics, P.O. Box 333, 836 N. La Cienega Blvd., West Hollywood, CA 90069. *We release issues erratically as compelling information appears, and are not on a strict schedule.*

Be sure to specify which issue you want to start with when you order. We suggest that you look over the contents of the back issues and consider ordering some of them as they cover many different subjects related to this approach. For a free sample issure, send us a request.

References

What Is AIDS-Related Wasting?

1. Anon. Muscle provides glutamine to the immune system. *Nutri Rev* (1990) 48:390-392.
2. Ardawi, MS, et al. Metabolism in lymphocytes and its importance in the immune response. *Essays in Biochem* (1985) 21:143.
3. Newsholme, EA. Psychoimmunology and cellular nutrition: an alternative hypothesis. *Biol Psychiat* (1990) 27:1-3.
4. Kotler, DP, et al. Magnitude of body-cell-mass depletion and the timing of death from wasting in AIDS. *Am J Clin Nutr* (1989) 50:444-447.

Wasting Syndrome Treatment Issues

1. Bucher, G, et al. A prospective study on the safety and effect of nandrolone decanoate in HIV-positive patients. XI International Conference on AIDS, Vancouver (1996) 11(1):26. Abstract No. Mo.B.423.
2. Schlumpberger, JM, et al. CD8 lymphocyte counts and the risk of death in advanced HIV infection. *J Fam Pract* (1994) 38(1):33-38.
3. Calabrese, LH, et al. The effects of anabolic steroids and strength training on the human immune response. *Med Sci Sports Exercise* (1989) 21(4):386-392.

Megace — The Wrong Drug

1. Spaulding, M. Anorexia and appetite stimulation in cancer patients. *Oncol* (1989) 3(suppl):17-23.
2. Wade, GN, et al. Theoretical review: gonadal effects on food intake and adiposity, a metabolic hypothesis. *Physiol Behav* (1979) 22:583-593.
3. Hervey, E, et al. Energy storage in female rats with progesterone in absence of increased food intake. *J Physiol* (1967) 200:118-119.
4. Oster, MH. Megestrol acetate in patients with AIDS. *Ann Int Med* (1994) 15;121(6):400-408.
5. Harte, C, et al. Progestagens and Cushing's syndrome. *Int J Med Sci* (1995) 165(4):274-275.
6. Hamburger, AW, et al. Megestrol acetate induced differentiation of 3T3-L1 adipocytes in vitro. *Semin Oncol* (1988) 15(suppl 1):76-78.
7. Summerbell, CD. Megestrol acetate vs cyproheptadine in the treatment of weight loss associated with HIV infection. *Int J STD AIDS* (1992) 3:278-280.
8. Furth, PA. Megestrol acetate and cachexia associated with human immunodeficiency virus infection (letter). *Ann Int Med* (1989) 110(8):667.

9. Henry, K, et al. Diabetes mellitus induced by megestrol acetate in a patient with AIDS and cachexia. *Ann Int Med* (1992) 116(1):53-54.

10. Von Roenn, JH, et al. Megestrol acetate for treatment of anorexia and cachexia associated with human immunodeficiency virus infection. *Sem Oncol* (1990) 17(suppl 9)(6):13-16.

11. DiSaia, PJ, et al. Unusual side effect of megestrol acetate. *Am J Obstet Gynecol* (1977) 15(4):460-461.

Biolectric Impedance Analysis (BIA) And AIDS Survival

1. Kotler, D, et al. Magnitude of body cell mass depletion and timing of death from wasting in AIDS. *Am J Clin Nutr* (1989) 50:444-447.

2. Muurahainen, N, et al. Detection of occult wasting by BIA technology. Graduate Hospital of Philadelphia. X International Conference on AIDS, Tokyo (1994) Aug 7-12; 10(2):220. Abstract No. PB0895.

3. Sluys, T, et al. Body composition in patients with acquired immunodeficiency syndrome: a validation study of bioelectrical impedance analysis. *J Parent Ent Nutr* (1993) 17(5):404-406.

4. Wang, J, et al. Body fat measurement in patients with acquired immunodeficiency syndrome: which method should be used? *Am J Clin Nutr* (1992) 56(6):963-967.

5. Jacobs, DO. Bioelectric impedance analysis: a way to assess changes in body cell mass in patients with AIDS? *J Parent Ent Nutr* (1993) 17(5):401-402.

Appetite Stimulation: Megace, Medicinal Marijuana, and Marinol

1. Denning, DW, et al. Pulmonary Aspergillosis in AIDS. *N Eng J Med* (1991) 324:654-662.

2. Tindall, B, et al. The Sidney AIDS Project: development of acquired immunodeficiency syndrome in a group of HIV seropositive homosexual men. *Aust N Z J Med* (1988) 18:8-15.

3. Caiffa, WT, et al. Drug smoking, *Pneumocystis carinii* pneumonia, and immunosuppression increase risk of bacterial pneumonia in human immunodeficiency virus-seropositive drug users. *Am J Respir Crit Care Med* (1994) 150:1493-1498.

4. Sherman, MP. Anti-microbial respiratory burst characteristics of pulmonary alveolar macrophages recovered from smokers of marijuana alone, smokers of tobacco alone, smokers of marijuana and tobacco, and nonsmokers. *Am Rev Respir Dis* (1991) 144.1351-1356.

5. Schwartz, RH, et al. Marijuana to prevent nausea and vomiting in cancer patients: a survey of clinical oncologists. *South Med J* (1997) 90(2):167-172.

6. Beal, JE, et al. Dronabinol as a treatment for anorexia associated with weight loss in patients with AIDS. *J Pain Sympt Man* (1995) 10:89-97.

How Do Anabolic Steroids Work?

1. Schulte-Beerbuhl, M, et al. Comparison of testosterone, dihydrotestosterone, luteinizing hormone, and follicle-stimulating hormone in serum after injection of testosterone enanthate or tesosterone cypionate. *Fert Steril* (1980) 33:201-203.

2. Nankin, HR. Hormone kinetics after intramuscular testosterone cypionate. *Fertil Steril* (1987) Jun; 47(6):1004-1009.

3. Bergink, EW, et al. Metabolism and receptor binding of nandrolone and testosterone under in vitro and in vivo conditions. *Acta Endocrinologica* (1985) 271 (suppl):31-37.

4. Vida, JA. *Androgens and Anabolic Agents.* Academic Press (NY/London) (1969):16.

5. Haupt, HA, et al. Anabolic steroids: a review of the literature. *Am J Sport Med* (1984) 12.6:469-484.

6. O'Shea, JP, et al. Biochemical and physical effects of an anabolic steroid in competi-

tive swimmers and weightlifters. *Nutr Rep Int* (1970) 2:351-362.

7. Kantor, MA, et al. Androgens reduce HDL2-cholesterol and increase hepatic triglyceride lipase activity. *Med Sci Sports Exerc* (1985) 17(4):462-465.

8. Berger, J, et al. Effect of anabolic steroids on HIV-related wasting. *So Med J* (1993) August 86(8):865-866.

9. Woodard, TL, et al. Glucose intolerance and insulin resistance in aplastic anemia treated with oxymetholone. *J Clin Endocrinol Metab* (1981) 53(5):905-908.

10. Wijnand, HP, et al. Pharmacokinetic parameters of nandrolone decanoate to healthy volunteers. *Acta Endocrinol Suppl* (Copenhagen) (1985) 271:19-30.

11. Welder, AA, et al. Toxic effects of anabolic-androgenic steroids in primary rat hepatic cell cultures. *J Pharmacol Toxicol Methods* (1995) 33(4):187-195.

12. Herzenberg, L, et al. Glutathione deficiency is associated with impaired survival in HIV disease. *Proceedings of the National Academy of Sciences* USA (1997) 94(5):1967-1972.

13. Salvato, P, et al., 2nd International Conference on Nutrition and HIV Infection, Cannes, France (1997) April 23-24; Abstract No. 0-003.

14. Wijnand, HP, et al. Pharmacokinetic parameters of nandrolone decanoate to healthy volunteers. *Acta Endocrinol Suppl* (Copenh) (1985) 271:19-30.

15. Gold, J, et al. Safety and efficacy of nandrolone decanoate for treatment of wasting in patients with HIV infection. *AIDS* (1996) 10(7):745-752.

16. Coodley, GO, et al. A trial of testosterone therapy for HIV-associated weight loss. *AIDS* (1997) 11(11):1347-1352.

17. Bhasin, S, et al. The effect of supraphysiological doses of testosterone on muscle size and strength in normal men. *N Engl J Med* (1996) Jul 4; 335(1):1-7.

18. Friedl, KE, et al. Comparison of the effects of high dose testosterone and 19-nortestosterone to a replacement dose of testosterone on strength and body composition in normal men. *J Steroid Biochem Mol Biol* (1991) 40(4-6):607-612.

19. Kurz, EM, et al. Androgens regulate the dendritic length of mammalian motoneurons in adulthood. *Science* (1986) 232:395-398.

20. Marquardt, GH, et al. Failure of non-17-alkylated steroids to produce abnormal liver function tests. *J Clin Endocrinol* (1964) 24:1334-1336.

21. Davignon, J, et al. Triglycerides: a risk factor for coronary heart disease. Atherosclerosis (1996) 124 Suppl():S57-64.

22. Lennon, HD, et al. Anabolic activity of 2-oxa-17alpha-methyldihydrotestosterone (oxandrolone) in castrated rats. *Steroids* (1964) 4:689-697.

23. Kochakian, CD. Personal communication to Michael Mooney, 1995.

24. Hengge, UR, et al. Oxymetholone promotes weight gain in patients with advanced human immunodeficiency virus infection. *Brit J Nutr* (1996) 75:129-138.

25. Beyler, AL, et al. Reversal by androstanozole of catabolic action of cortisone acetate. 1st International Congress on Endocrinology, Copenhagen Advanced Abstracts of Short Communications (Fuchs, F. ed) *Periodica* (1960) p. 829

26. Harding, HR, et al. The anti-catabolic activity of anabolic steroids based on the suppression of cortisone acetate (EAc) induction of liver tryptophan pyrrolase. VI th Pan American Congress on Endocinology, Mexico (1965).

27. Thacker, DL, et al., Metabolism of an anabolic androgenic steroid oxymetholone by human cytochrome P450s. *Clin Pharmacol Ther* (1999) 65(2):136 Abstract PI-75.

First Placebo-Controlled Steroid Study Suggests Improved Immune Function

1. Kotler, DP, et al. Magnitude of body-cell-mass depletion and the timing of death from wasting in AIDS. *Am J Clin Nutr* (1989) 50:444-447.

2.. Schlumpberger, JM, et al. CD8 lymphocyte counts and the risk of death in advanced HIV infection. *J Fam Pract* (1994) 38(1):33-38.

Steroid Legality and The Physician

1. Coodley, GO, et al. A trial of testosterone therapy for HIV-associated weight loss. *AIDS* (1997) 11(11):1347-1352.
2. Rabkin, JG, et al. Testosterone replacement therapy in HIV illness. *Gen Hosp Psychiat* (1995) Jan;17(1):37-42.
3. Dobs, AS, et al. Endocrine disorders in men infected with human immunodeficiency virus. *Am J Med* (1988) 84(3, Pt 2):611-616
4. Kotler, DP, et al. Magnitude of body-cell-mass depletion and the timing of death from wasting in AIDS. *Am J Clin Nutr* (1989) 50:444-447.
5. Grinspoon, SC, et al. Body composition and endocrine function in women with acquired immunodeficiency syndrome wasting. *J Clin Endocrinol Metab* (1997) 82(5):1332-1337.

An Initiative: New Directions for Wasting Research from Program for Wellness Restoration (PoWeR)

1. Berger, D, et al. Measurement of Body Weight and Body Cell Mass in Patients receiving Highly Active Antiretroviral Therapy (HAART). *Proceedings ICAAC Conference, Toronto* (1997) October.
2. Jeantils, V, et al. Weight gain under oral testosterone undecanoate in AIDS. *Therapie* (1993) 48:59-72.
3. Berger, J, et al. Effect of anabolic steroids on HIV-related wasting myopathy. *So Med J* (1993) August; 86(8):865-866.
4. Rabkin, JG, et al. Testosterone replacement therapy in HIV illness. *Gen Hosp Psychiatry* (1995) 17(1):37-42.
5. Dobs, AS, et al. Endocrine disorders in men infected with human immunodeficiency virus. *Am J Med* (1988) 84(3, pt 2):611-616.

6. Gilden, D. Anabolic steroids for wasting. Interview with Dr. Barry Chadsey. *AIDS Treatment News* (1993) #187;4.
7. Jekot, W, et al. Treating HIV/AIDS patients with anabolic steroids. *AIDS Patient Care* (1993) 3:68-74.
8. Bhasin, S, et al. The effect of supraphysiological doses of testosterone on muscle size and strength in normal men. *N Engl J Med* (1996) 335(1):1-7.
9. Gold, J, et al. Safety and efficacy of nandrolone decanoate for treatment of wasting in patients with HIV infection. *AIDS* (1996) 10(7):745-752.
10. Bucher, G, et al. A prospective study on the safety and effect of nandrolone decanoate in HIV-positive patients. XI International Conference on AIDS, Vancouver (1996) 11(1):26. Abstract No. Mo.B.423.
11. Strawford, A, et al. Effects of nandrolone decanoate (ND) on nitrogen balance, metabolism, body composition and function in men with AIDS wasting syndrome (AWS). 2nd International Conference on Nutrition and HIV Infection, Cannes, France (1997):267.
12. Hengge, UR, et al. Oxymetholone promotes weight gain in patients with advanced human immunodeficiency virus infection. *Brit J of Nutr* (1996) 75:129-138.
13. Ott, M, et al. Biolectrical impedance analysis as a predictor of survival in patients with human immunodeficiency virus infection. *J Acquir Immune Def Synd Hum Retro.* (1995) 9(1):20-25.
14. Li, ZG, et al. Effects of gonadal steroids on the production of IL-1 and IL-6 by blood mononuclear cells in vitro. *Clin and Exp Rheum* (1993) 11(2):157-162.
15. Klein, SA, et al. Substitution of testosterone in a HIV positive patient with hypogonadism and wasting syndrome led to a reduced rate of apoptosis. *Eur J Med Res* (1997) 2(1):30-32.

16. Wagner, G, et al. Illness stage, concurrent medications, and other correlates of low testosterone in men with HIV. *J AIDS Hum Retro* (1995) 8(2):204-207.

17. Salvato, P, et al., 2nd International Conference on Nutrition and HIV Infection, Cannes, France (1997) April 23-24; Abstract No. 0-003.

18. Strawford, A, et al. Resistance exercise and supraphysiologic androgen therapy in eugonadal men with HIV-related weight loss. *JAMA* (1999) 281(14):1282-1290.

19. Sattler, F, et al. Effects of Pharmacological Doses of Nandrolone Decanoate and Progressive Resistance Training in Immunodeficient Patients Infected with Human Immunodeficiency Virus. *J Clin Endo Metabol* (1999) 84(4):1268-1276.

Complementary Approaches To Treating Lipodystrophy

1. Karnieli, E, et al. Insulin resistance in Cushing's syndrome. *Horm Metab Res* (1985) 17(10):518-521.

2. Oehler, G, et al. Hyperinsulinaemia and impaired glucose tolerance in chronic inflammatory liver disease (author's disease). *Z Gastroenterol* (1981) 19(1):26-32.

3. Laakso, M, Insulin resistance and coronary heart disease. *Curr Opin Lipidol* (1996) 7(4):217-226.

4. Björntorp, P. The regulation of adipose tissue distribution in humans. *Int J Obes Relat Metab Disord* (1996) 20(4):291-302.

5. Haffner, SM. Decreased testosterone and dehydroepiandrosterone sulfate concentrations are associated with increased insulin and glucose concentrations in nondiabetic men. *Metabol* (1994) 43(5):599-603.

6. Marcelli, JM, et al. Female obesity: testosterone is positively correlated with peripheral insulin resistance. *Ann Endocrinol* (Paris) (1993) 54(3):169-173.

7. Armellini, F, et al. Interrelationships between intraabdominal fat and total serum testosterone levels in obese women. *Metabolism* (1994) 43(3):390-5.

8. Benbrik, E, et al. Cellular and mitochondrial toxicity of zidovudine (AZT) didanosine (ddI) and zalcitabine (ddC) on cultured human muscle cells. *J Neurol Sci* (1997) 149(1):19-25.

9. Kotler, DP, et al. Magnitude of body-cell-mass depletion and the timing of death from wasting in AIDS. *Am J Clin Nutr* (1989) 50:444-447.

10. Greene, JB, et al. Clinical approach to weight loss in the patient with HIV infections. *Gastro Clinics of No Amer* (1988) 17(3):573-576.

11. Hellerstein, MK, et al. Increased de novo hepatic lipogenesis in human immunodeficiency virus infection. *J Clin Endocrinol Metab* (1993) 76(3):559-565.

12. Grinspoon, SC, et al. Loss of lean body and muscle mass correlates with androgen levels in hypogonadal men with acquired immunodeficiency syndrome and wasting. *J Clin Endocrinol Metab* (1996) 81(11):4051-4058.

13. Grinspoon, SC, et al. Body composition and endocrine function in women with acquired immunodeficiency syndrome wasting. *J Clin Endocrinol Metab* (1997) 82(5):1332-1337.

14. Parsch, CJ, et al. Injectable testosterone undecanoate has more favourable pharmacokinetics and pharmacodynamics than testosterone enanthate. *Euro J of Endo* (1995) 132:514-519.

15. Rabkin, JG, et al. Testosterone replacement therapy for HIV-infected men. *The AIDS Reader* (1995) July/August:136-144.

16. Marin, P, et al. Androgen replacement of middle aged, obese men: effects on metabolism, muscle, and adipose tissues. *Eur J Med* (1992) 1(6):329-336.

17. Henricksson, J, et al. Influence of exercise on insulin sensitivity. *J Cardio Risk* (1995) 2(4):303-309.

18. McCarty, MF, et al. Reduction of free fatty acids may ameliorate risk factors associated with abdominal obesity. *Med Hypotheses* (1995) 44(4):278-286.

19. Truswell, AS. Food carbohydrates and plasma lipids — an update. *Am J Clin Nutr* (1994) 59(suppl)(3):S710S-3718.

20. Miller, JC, ct al. Replacing starch with sucrose in a high glycaemic index breakfast cereal lowers glycaemic and insulin responses. *Eur J Clin Nutr* (1994) 48(10):749-752.

21. Wilson, BE, et al. Effects of chromium supplementation on fasting insulin levels and lipid parameters in healthy, non-obese young subjects. *Diabetes Res Clin Pract* (1995) 28(3):179-184.

22. Anderson, RA, et al. Elevated intake of supplemental chromium improves glucose and insulin variables in individuals with type 2 diabetes. *Diabetes* (1997) 46:1786-1791.

23. Jacobs, S, et al. Enhancement of glucose disposal in patients with type 2 diabetes by alpha-lipoic acid. *Drug Res* (1995) 45:872-874.

24. Estrada, EH, et al. Stimulation of glucose uptake by the natural coenzyme a-lipoic acid/thioctic acid. *Diabetes* (1996) 45:1798-1804.

25. Busse, E, et al. Influence of alpha-lipoic acid on intracellular glutathione in vitro and in vivo. *Arzneimittel-Forshung* (1992) 42:829-831.

26. Herzenberg L, et al. Glutathione deficiency is associated with impaired survival in IIIV disease. *Proceedings of the National Academy of Sciences USA* (1997) 94(5):1967-1972.

27. De Simone, C, et al. High dose L-carnitine improves immunologic and metabolic parameters in AIDS patients. *Immunopharmacol Immunotoxicol* (1993) 15(1):1-12.

28. Hellerstein, MK, et al. Effects of dietary n-3 fatty acid supplementation in men with weight loss associated with the acquired immune deficiency syndrome: Relation to indices of cytokine production. *J AIDS Hum Retro* (1996)11(3):258-270.

29. Faure, P, et al. Vitamin E improves the free radical defense system potential and insulin sensitivity of rats fed high fructose diets. *J Nutr* (1997) 127(1):103-107.

30. Basualdo, CG, et al. Vitamin A (retinol) status of first nation adults with non-insulin-dependent diabetes mellitus. *J Am Coll Nutr* (1997) 16(1):39-45.

31. Mak, RH, et al. The vitamin D/parathyroid hormone axis in the pathogenesis of hypertension and insulin resistance in uremia. *Miner Electrolyte Metab* (1992) 18(2-5): 156-159.

32. Sanchez, M, et al. Oral calcium supplementation reduces intraplatelet free calcium concentration and insulin resistance in essential hypertensive patients. *Hypertension* (1997) 29(1 Pt 2):531-536.

33. Facchini, F, et al. Relation between dietary vitamin intake and resistance to insulin-mediated glucose disposal in healthy volunteers. *Am J Clin Nutr* (1996) 63(6):946-949.

34. Hickson, RC, et al. Glutamine prevents down regulation of myosin heavy chain synthesis and muscle atrophy from glucocorticoids. *Am J Physiol [Endo Metab]* (1995) 269(31):E730-E734.

35. Hong, RW, et al. Glutamine preserves liver glutathione after lethal hepatic injury. *Ann Surg* (1992) 215(2):114-119.

36. Bounous, G, et al. Whey protein as a food supplement in HIV-seropositive individuals. *Clin Invest Med* (1993) 16(3):204-209.

37. Guthrie, R. Treatment of non-insulin-dependent diabetes mellitus with metformin. *J Am Board Fam Pract* (1997) 10(3):213-221.

38. Engelson, ES, et al. Nutrition and testosterone status in HIV-positive women. XI International Conference on AIDS, Vancouver (1996) Abstract Tu. B.2382.

39. Laudat, A, et al. Changes in systemic gonadal and adrenal steroids in asymptomatic human immunodeficiency virus-infected men: relationship with the CD4 cell counts. *Eur J Endocrinol* (1995) 133(4):418-424.

40. Friedl, KE, et al. The administration of pharmacological doses of testosterone or 19-nortestosterone to normal men is not associated with increased insulin secretion or impaired glucose tolerance. *J Clin Endocrinol Metab* (1989) May 68(5):971-5.

41. Velussi, M, et al. Long-term (12 months) treatment with an antioxidant drug (silymarin) is effective on hyperinsulinemia, exogenous insulin need and malondialdehyde levels in cirrhotic diabetic patients. *J of Hepatol* (1997) 26:871-879.

42. Martin, ME, et al. Alterations in the concentrations and binding properties of sex steroid binding protein and corticosteroid-binding globulin in HIV-positive patients. *J Endocrinol Invest* (1992) 15(8):597-603.

43. Peterson, JC, et al. Vitamins and progression of atherosclerosis in hyperhomocysteinemia. *Lancet* (1998) Jan 24, 351(9098):263.

44. Woodard, TL, et al. Glucose intolerance and insulin resistance in aplastic anemia treated with oxymetholone. *J Clin Endocrinol Metab* (1981) 53(5):905-908.

46. Devara, JS, et al. The effects of alpha tocopherol supplementation on monocyte function. Decreased lipid oxidation interleukin 1 beta secretion and monocyte adhesion to endothelium. *J Clin Invest* (1996) 98(3):756-763.

47. Munoz, JA, et al. Effect of vitamin C on lipoproteins in healthy adults. *Ann Med Interne (Paris)* (1994) 145(1):13-19.

48. Refsum, H, et al. Homocysteine and cardiovascular disease. *Annu Rev Med* (1998) 49:31-62.

49. Haffner, SM. Sex hormone-binding protein, hyperinsulinemia, insulin resistance and noninsulin-dependent diabetes. *Horm Res* (1996) 45(3-5):233-237.

50. Moller, J. *Cholesterol: Interactions with Testosterone and Cortisol in Cardiovascular Disease,* Springer-Verlag; Berlin (1987).

51. Pamies-Andreu, E, et al. High-fructose feeding elicits insulin resistance without hypertension in normal mongrel dogs. *Am J Hypertens* (1995) 8(7):732-738.

52. Liu, S, et al. Dietary omega-3 and polyunsaturated fatty acids modify fatty acid composition and insulin binding in skeletal-muscle sarcolemma. *Biochem J* (1994) 299 (pt 3):831-837.

53. Baum, M, et al. Inadequate dietary intake and altered nutrition status in early HIV-1 infection. *Nutrition* (1994) 10(1):16-20.

54. Baum, MK, et al. Micronutrients and HIV-1 disease progression. *AIDS* (1995) 9(9):1051-1056.

55. Chen, YD, et al. Why do low-fat high-carbohydrate diets accentuate postprandial lipemia in patients with NIDDM? *Diabetes Care* (1995) 18(1):10-16.

56. Torres, RA, et al. Treatment of dorsocervical fat pads (buffalo hump) and truncal obesity with Serostim (recombinant human growth hormone) in patients with AIDS maintained on HAART. XII International AIDS Conference, Geneva (1998) June 28-July 3. Abstract No. 32164.

57. Kantor, MA, et al. Androgens reduce HDL2-cholesterol and increase hepatic triglyceride lipase activity. *Med Sci Sports Exerc* (1985) 17(4):462-5.

58. Kailin, X, et al. Hyperinsulinemia accompanying hyperglycemia in Chinese patients with aplastic anemia. *Am J Hematol* (1997) 56(3):151-4.

59. Applebaum-Bowden D, et al. The dyslipoproteinemia of anabolic steroid therapy: increase in hepatic triglyceride lipase precedes the decrease in high-density lipoprotein 2 cholesterol. *Metab* (1987) 36(10):949-952.

60. Dieterich, D, et al. Incidence of body habitus changes in a cohort of 700 HIV-infected patients. *Infect Diseases Soc Amer* (1998) Nov 12 - 15. Abstract No. 477.

61. Mulligan, KE, et al. Evidence of unique metabolic effects of protease inhibitors. 5th Conf Retrovir Oppor Infect (1998) Feb 1-5;157 (Abstract No. 414).

62. Walli, RK, et al. Peripheral insulin resistance leading to impaired glucose tolerance in HIV-1 infected patients treated with pro-

tease inhibitors. Int Conf AIDS, Geneva (1998)12:777 (Abstract No. 179/41177).

63. Carr, A, et al. Pathogenesis of HIV-1 protease inhibitor-associated periperal lipodystrophy, hyperlipidaemia, and insulin resistance. *Lancet* (1998) Jun 20;351(9119):1881-1883.

64. Saint-Marc, T, et al. Metformin (Glucophage®) Poster 672, 6th Retrovirus Conference, Chicago (1999) Feb.

65. Ponte, E, et al. Cardiovascular disease and omega-3 fatty acids. *Minerva Med* (1997) 88(9):343-53.

66. Mori, TA, et al. Interactions between dietary fat, fish, and fish oils and their effects on platelet function in men at risk of cardiovascular disease. *Arterioscler Thromb Vasc Biol* (1997) 17(2):279-286.

67. Nadler, JL, et al. Magnesium deficiency produces insulin resistance and increased thromboxane synthesis. *Hypertension* (1993) 21(6 Pt 2):1024-1029.

68. Storlien, LH, et al. Influence of dietary fat composition on development of insulin resistance in rats. Relationship to muscle triglyceride and omega-3 fatty acids in muscle phospholipid. *Diabetes* (1991) 40(2):280-289.

69. Berry, EM. Dietary fatty acids in the management of diabetes mellitus. *Am J Clin Nutr* (1997) 66(4 Suppl):991S-997S.

70. Yam, D, et al. Diet and disease—the Israeli paradox: possible dangers of a high omega-6 polyunsaturated fatty acid diet. *Isr J Med Sci* (1996) 32(11):1134-1143.

71. Lemon, PW, et al. Do athletes need more dietary protein and amino acids? *Int J Sports Nutri* (1995) 5:S39-S61.

72. Lemon, PW, et al. Protein requirements and muscle mass strength changes during intensive training in novice bodybuilders. *J Appl Physiol* (1992) 73(2):767-775.

73. Boirie, Y, et al. Slow and fast dietary proteins differently modulate postprandial protein accretion. Proceedings of the National Academy of Science USA (1997) 94: 14930-14935.

74. Reddi, A, et al. Biotin supplementation improves glucose and insulin tolerances in genetically diabetic KK mice. *Life Sci* (1988) 42(13):1323-1330.

75. Koutsikos, D, et al. Oral glucose tolerance test after high-dose i.v. biotin administration in normoglucemic hemodialysis patients. *Ren Fail* (1996) 18(1):131-137.

76. Koutsikos D, et al. Biotin for diabetic peripheral neuropathy. *Biomed Pharmacother* (1990) 44(10):511-514.

77. Sheard, NF. The diabetic diet: evidence for a new approach. *Nutr Rev* (1995) 53(1):16-18.

78. Garg, A, et al. Effects of varying carbohydrate content of diet in patients with non-insulin-dependent diabetes mellitus [see comments] *JAMA* (1994) 271(18):1421-1428.

79. Ascherio, A, et al. Health effects of trans fatty acids. *Am J Clin Nutr* (1997) 66(4 Suppl):1006S-1010S.

80. Hobbs, CJ, et al. Nandrolone, a 19-nortestosterone, enhances insulin-independent glucose uptake in normal men. [see comments] *J Clin Endocrinol Metab* (1996) 81(4):1582-1585.

81. O'Neal, DN, et al. The effect of 3 months of recombinant human growth hormone (GH) therapy on insulin and glucose-mediated glucose disposal and insulin secretion in GH-deficient adults: a minimal model analysis. *J Clin Endocrinol Metab* (1994) 79(4):975-983.

82. Móldrup, A, et al. Multiple growth hormone-binding proteins are expressed on insulin-producing cells. *Mol Endocrinol* (1989) 3(8):1173-1182.

83. Opara, EC, et al. L-glutamine supplementation of a high fat diet reduces body weight and attenuates hyperglycemia and hyperinsulinemia in C57BL/6J mice. *J Nutr* (1996) 126(1):273-279.

84. Borel, MJ, et al. Parenteral glutamine infusion alters insulin-mediated glucose metabolism. *J Parenter Enteral Nutr* (1998) 22(5):280-285.

85. Tatsuhiro, M, et al., et al. Beef tallow diet decreases lipoprotein lipase activities in

brown adipose tissue, heart, and soleus muscle in reducing sympathetic activities in rats. *J Nutr Sci Vitaminol* (1994) 40:569-581.

86. Okuno M, et al., Perilla oil prevents the excessive growth of visceral adipose tissue in rats by down-regulating adipocyte differentiation. *J Nutr* (1997) 127(9):1752-1757.

87. Bolinder, J, et al., Site differences in insulin receptor binding and insulin action in subcutaneous fat of obese females. *J Clin Endocr Metab* (1983) 57:455-461.

88. Bruning, PF, et al., Insulin resistance and breast-cancer risk. *Int J Cancer* (1992) 52(4):511-516.

89. Singh, PN, et al., Dietary risk factors for colon cancer in a low-risk population. *Am J Epidemiol* (1998) 148(8):761-774.

90. Gerber, M. Energy balance and cancers. *Eur J Cancer Prev* (1999) 8(2):77-89.

91. Banerji, MA, et al., Body composition, visceral fat, leptin, and insulin resistance in Asian Indian men. *J Clin Endocrinol Metab* (1999) 84(1):137-144.

Can Switching Anti-Retroviral Drugs Reduce Lipodystrophy?

1. Martinez, E, et al., Reversion of metabolic abnormalities after switching from HIV-1 protease inhibitors to nevirapine. AIDS (1999) 13:805-810.

2. Moyle, G, et al., Management of Indinavir-associated metabolic changes by substitution with Efavirenz in virologically controlled HIV+ persons. Sixth Retrovirus Conference, Chicago (1999) Feb. Abstract No. 668.

Anabolic Steroids—Adverse Effects Rumors and Realities

1. Thompson, PD, et al. Contrasting effects of testosterone and stanozolol on serum lipoprotein levels. *J Am Med Assoc* (1989) 261(8):1165-1168.

2. Glazer, G., et al. Lack of demonstrated effect of nandrolone on serum lipids. *Metabolism* (1994) 43(2):204-210.

3. Hara, T, et al. Oxandrolone and plasma triglyceride reduction: effect on triglyceride-rich and high density lipoproteins. *Artery* (1981) 9(5):328-341.

4. Reeves, RD, et al. Hyperlipidemia due to oxymetholone therapy. Occurrence in a long-term hemodialysis patient. *J Am Med Assoc* (1976) 236(5):469-472.

5. Zgliczynski, S, et al. Effect of testosterone replacement therapy on lipids and lipoproteins in hypogonadal and elderly men. *Atherosclerosis* (1996) 121(1):35-43.

6. Hanash, KA, et al. Androgen effect on prostate specific antigen secretion. *J Surg Oncol* (1992) 49(3):202-204.

7. Svetec, DA, et al. The effect of parenteral testosterone replacement on prostate specific antigen in hypogonadal men with erectile dysfunction. *J Urol* (1997) 158(5):1775-1777.

8. Douglas, TH, et al. Effect of exogenous testosterone replacement on prostate-specific antigen and prostate-specific membrane antigen levels in hypogonadal men. *J Surg Oncol* (1995) 59(4):246-250.

9. Gann, PH, et al. Prospective study of sex-hormone levels and risk of prostate cancer. *J Natl Cancer Inst* (1996) 88(16):1118-1126.

10. Ribeiro, M, et al. Low serum testosterone and a younger age predict for a poor outcome in metastatic prostate cancer. *Am J Clin Oncol* (1997) 20(6):605-608.

11. Monda, LM, et al. The correlation between serum prostate-specific antigen and prostate cancer is not influenced by the serum testosterone concentration. *Urology* (1995) 46(1):62-64.

12. Rabkin, JG, et al. Testosterone treatment of clinical hypogonadism in patients with HIV/AIDS. *Int J STD AIDS* (1997) 8:537-545.

13. Suzuki, K, et al. Endocrine environment of benign prostatic hyperplasia: prostate size and volume are correlated with serum estrogen concentration. *Scand J Urol Nephrol* (1995) 29:65-68.

14. Gann, PH, et al. A prospective study of plasma hormone levels, nonhormonal factors, and development of benign prostatic hyperplasia. *The Prostate* (1995) 26:40-49.

15. Marquardt, GH, et al. Failure of non-17-alkylated steroids to produce abnormal liver function tests. *J Clin Endocrinol* (1964) 24:1334-1336.

16. Welder, AA, et al. Toxic effects of anabolic-androgenic steroids in primary rat hepatic cell cultures. *J Pharmacol Toxicol Methods* (1995) 33(4):187-195.

17. Hickson, RC, et al., Adverse effects of anabolic steroids. *Med Toxicol Adv Drug Exp* (1989) 4:254-271.

18. Ishak, KG, et al., Hepatotoxic effects of the anabolic/androgenic steroids. *Semin Liver Dis* (1987) 7(3):230-236.

19. Kosaka, A, et al., Hepatocellular carcinoma associated with anabolic steroid therapy: report of a case and review of the Japanese literature. *J Gastroenterol* (1996) 31(3):450-454.

20. Hernandez-Nieto, L, et al., Benign liver-cell adenoma associated with long-term administration of an androgenic-anabolic steroid (methandienone). *Cancer* (1977) 40(4):1761-1764.

Anabolic Hormones — Adverse Effects And Remedies

1. Metzger, DL, et al. Estrogen receptor blockade with tamoxifen diminishes growth hormone secretion in boys: evidence for a stimulatory role of endogenous estrogens during male adolescence. *J Clin Endocrinol Metab* (1994) 79(2):513-518.

2. el-Sheikh, MM, et al. The effect of Permixon (saw palmetto) on androgen receptors. *J Acta Obstet Gynecol Scand* (1988) 67(5):397-399.

3. Suzuki, K, et al. Endocrine environment of benign prostatic hyperplasia: prostate size and volume are correlated with serum estrogen concentration. *Scand J Urol Nephrol* (1995) 29:65-68.

4. Gann, PH, et al. A prospective study of plasma hormone levels, nonhormonal factors, and development of benign prostatic hyperplasia. *The Prostate* (1995) 26:40-49.

Anabolic Steroids and Kaposi's Sarcoma

1. Trattner, A, et al. The appearance of Kaposi's sarcoma during corticosteroid therapy. *Cancer* (1993) Sep. 1; 72(5):1779-1783.

2. Guo, W, et al. Increased levels of glucocorticoid receptors (GR) expression in AIDS-Kaposi's sarcoma. *Meeting Abstract. Proceedings of the Annual Meeting of the American Association of Cancer Research* (1993) 34:A3016.

3. Schulhafer, EP, et al. Steroid-induced Kaposi's sarcoma in a patient with pre-AIDS. *Am J Med* (1987) Feb:82(2): 313-317.

4. Martin, RW, et al. Kaposi's Sarcoma. *Medicine* (1993)72:245-261.

5. Rosenthal, E, et al. Estrogen, progesterone, and androgen and their receptors in epidemic Kaposi's sarcoma. IX International Conference on AIDS, Berlin (1993) Jun 6-11; 9(1):403. Abstract No. PO-B12-1605.

6. Christeff, N, et al. Differences in androgens of HIV positive with and without KS. *East Parisian CISIH Group.* International Conference on AIDS, Berlin (1993) Jun 6-11; 9(1):400. Abstract No. PO-B12-1588.

7. Klauke, S, et al. Sex hormone as a cofactor in the pathogenesis of the epidemic of Kaposi's sarcoma. *AIDS* (1995) 9(11):1295-1296.

8. Shoefer, H, et al. Kaposi's sarcoma (HIV-positive and HIV) in caucasian women. International Conference on AIDS, Berlin (1993) Jun 6-11; 9(1):397. Abstract No. PO-B12-1569.

9. Lunardi, IY, et al. Tumorigenesis and metastasis of neoplastic KS cell lines in immunodeficient mice blocked by a human pregnancy hormone. *Nature* (1995) May 4; 375(652):64-68.

10. *Positively Aware*, July/August,1995:8.

Steroid For AIDS Therapy: A Comparison Table

1. Ooshika, N, et al. Effect of an anabolic steroid on cellular immunity and postoperative evaluation of uterine cervical cancer. *Jap J of Canc Chemo* (1984) 11(10):2177-2184.

2. Mendenhall, CL, et al. Anabolic steroid effects on immune function: differences between analogues. *J Ster Biochem Molec Biol* (1990) 37(1):71-76.

3. Marquardt, GH, et al. Failure of non-17-alkylated steroids to produce abnormal liver function tests. *J Clin Endocrinol* (1964) 24:1334-1336.

4. Kotler, DP, et al. Magnitude of body-cell-mass depletion and the timing of death from wasting in AIDS. *Am J Clin Nutr* (1989) 50:444-447.

5. Calabrese, LH, et al. The effect of anabolic steroids and strength training on the human immune system. *Med Sci Sports Exerc* (1989) 21(4):386-392.

6. Huys, JV, et al. Effect of nandrolone decanoate on T-Cell lymphocytes during radiotherapy. *Clin Therap* (1979) 2(5):352-357.

7. Ansar, AS, et al. Sex hormones, immune responses, and autoimmune diseases. Mechanisms of sex hormone action. *Am J Pathol* (1985) 121(3):531-551.

8. Ehriches, L. Testosterone may prevent AIDS wasting. *Fam Pract* (1994) Oct. 10:36.

9. Jekot, WF, et al. Treating HIV/AIDS patients with anabolic steroids. *AIDS Patient Care* (1993) April; 7(2):11-17.

10. Gilden, D. Weight loss: a role for growth hormone and anabolic steroids. *AIDS Treatment News* (1993) Nov 19; 187:16.

11. Haupt, HA, et al. Anabolic steroids: a review of the literature. *Am J Sports Med* (1984) 12(6):469- 484.

12. Dickerman, RD, et al., Anabolic steroid-induced hepatotoxicity: is it overstated? *Clin J Sport Med* (1999) 9(1):34-39.

13. Welder, AA, et al. Toxic effects of anabolic-androgenic steroids in primary rat hepatic cell cultures. *J Pharmacol Toxicol Meth* (1995) 33(4):187-195.

14. Bucher, G, et al. A prospective study on the safety and effect of nandrolone decanoate in HIV-positive patients. XI International Conference on AIDS, Vancouver (1996) 11(1):26. Abstract No. Mo.B.423.

PoWeR Anabolic Hormone Guidelines

1. Ooshika, N, et al. Effect of an anabolic steroid on cellular immunity and postoperative evaluation of uterine cervical cancer. *Jap J of Canc Chemo* (1984) 11(10):2177-2184.

2. Calabrese, LH, et al. The effect of anabolic steroids and strength training on the human immune system. *Med Sci Sports Exerc* (1989) Aug; 21(4):386-392.

3. Huys, JV, et al. Effect of nandrolone decanoate on T-cell lymphocytes during radiotherapy. *Clin Ther* (1979) 2(5):352-357.

4. Plum, J. Influence of nandrolone decanoate on the repopulation of the thymus after total body irradiation of mice. *Immunopharm* (1982) 5:19.

5. Ansar, AS, et al. Sex hormones, immune responses, and autoimmune diseases. Mechanisms of sex hormone action. *Am J Pathol* (1985) Dec; 121(3):531-551.

6. Ahmed, SA, et al. Sex hormones and the immune system. *Ballieres Clinic Rheumat* (1990) Apr; 4(1):13-31.

7. Gilden, D. Weight loss: a role for growth hormone and anabolic steroids. *AIDS Treatment News* (1993) Nov 19; 187:16.

8. Mendenhall, CL, et al. Short-term and long-term survival in patients with alcoholic hepatitis treated with oxandrolone and prednisolone. *N Engl J Med* (1984) 311: 1464-1470.

9. Sundatam, K, et al. Different patterns of metabolism determine the relative anabolic

activity of 19-norandrogens. *J Ster Biochem Mol Biol* (1995) Jun; 53(1-6):253-257.

10. Vida, JA. *Androgens and Anabolic Agents.* Academic Press (NY/London) (1969):16.

11. Mendenhall, CL, et al. Anabolic steroid effects on immune function: differences between analogues. *J Steroid Biochem Molec Biol* (1990) 37(1):71-76.

12. Wijnand, HP, et al. Pharmacokinetic parameters of nandrolone decanoate to healthy volunteers. *Acta Endocrinol Suppl* (Copenh) (1985) 271:19-30.

13. Schulte-Beerbuhl, M, et al. Comparison of testosterone, dihydrotestosterone, luteinizing hormone, and follicle-stimulating hormone in serum after injection of testosterone enanthate or tesosterone cypionate. *Fert Steril* (1980) 33:201-203.

14. Nankin, HR, Hormone kinetics after intramuscular testosterone cypionate. *Fertil Steril* (1987) Jun; 47(6):1004-1009.

15. Berger, JR, et al. Effect of anabolic steroids on HIV-related wasting myopathy. *So Med J* (1993) Aug; 86(8):865-866.

16. Sinnecker, G, et al. Sex hormone-binding globulin response to the anabolic steroid stanozolol: evidence for its suitability as a biological androgen sensitivity test. *J Clin Endocrinol Metab* (1989) 68(6):1195-1200.

17. Beyler, AL, et al. Reversal by androstanozole of catabolic actions of cortisone acetate. First International Congress on Endocrinology, Copenhagen; Advanced Abstracts of Short Communications. *Periodica* (1960):829.

18. Metzger, DL, et al. Estrogen receptor blockade with tamoxifen diminishes growth hormone secretion in boys: evidence for a stimulatory role of endogenous estrogens during male adolescence. *J Clin Endocrinol Metab* (1994) 79(2):513-518.

19. Mendenhall, CL, et al. A study of oral nutritional support with oxandrolone in malnourished patients with alcoholic hepatitis: results of a Department of Veterans Affairs cooperative study. *Hepatology* (1993) 17(4):564-576.

20. Lovejoy, JC, et al. Oral anabolic steroid treatment, but not parental androgen treatment, decreases abdominal fat in obese, older men. *Int. J of Obesity* (1995) 19:614-624.

21. Krentz, AJ, et al. Anthropometric, metabolic, and immunological effects of recombinant human growth hormone in AIDS and AIDS-related complex. *J AIDS* (1993) 6:245-251.

22. Ott, M, et al. Bioelectrical impedance analysis as a predictor of survival in patients with human immunodeficiency virus infection. *J AIDS Hum Retro* (1995) 9:20-25.

23. Bounous, G, et al. Whey protein as a food supplement in HIV-seropositive individuals. *Clin Invest Med* (1993) Jun; 16(3):204-209.

24. Bounous, G, et al. Immunoenhancing property of dietary whey protein in mice: role of glutathione. *Clin Invest Med* (1989) 12:154-161.

25. Bounous, G, et al. The biological activity of undenatured dietary whey proteins: the role of glutathione. *Clin Invest Med* (1991) 14(4):296-309.

26. Ardawi, MS, et al. Glutamine metabolism in lymphocytes and its importance in the immune response. *Essays in Biochemistry* (1985).

27. Anon., Muscle provides glutamine to the immune system. *Nutrition Rev.* (1990) 48:390-392.

28. Mulligan, K, et al. Anabolic effects of recombinant human growth hormone in patients with wasting associated with human immunodeficiency virus infection. *J Clin Endocrinol Metab* (1993) 77(4):956-962.

29. Solerte, SB, et al. Hormonal and chronobiological impairment of GH-IGF1-IGFBP3 axis in HIV infected patients (CDC C3) with wasting syndrome. Effects of treatment with recombinant human GH. XI International AIDS Conference, Vancouver (1996) Abstract No. Mo. B.420.

30. Stoll, BA. Breast cancer risk in Japanese women with special reference to the growth

hormone-insulin-like growth factor axis. *Jpn J Clin Oncol* (1992) Feb; 22(1):1-5.

31. Westley, BR, et al. Role of insulin-like growth factors in steroid modulated proliferation. *J Ster Biochem Mol Biol* (1994) Oct; 51(1-2):1-9.

32. Kotler, DP, et al. Magnitude of body-cell-mass depletion and the timing of death from wasting in AIDS. *Am J Clin Nutr* (1989) 50:444-447.

33. Schlumpberger, JM, et al. CD8 lymphocyte counts and the risk of death in advanced HIV infection. *J of Fam Pract* (1994) 38(1):33-38.

34. Lennon, HD, et al. Anabolic activity of 2-oxa-17alpha-methyldihydrotestosterone (oxandrolone) in castrated rats. *Steroids* (1964) 4:689-697.

35. Beyler, AL, et al. Reversal by androstanozole of catabolic action of cortisone acetate. 1st International Congress on Endocrinology, Copenhagen Advanced Abstracts of Short Communications (Fuchs, F. ed) *Periodica* (1960) p. 829.

36. Harding, HR, et al. The anti-catabolic activity of anabolic steroids based on the suppression of cortisone acetate (EAc) induction of liver tryptophan pyrrolase. VI th Pan American Congress on Endocinology, Mexico (1965).

37. Mahesh, VB, et al. *Acta Endocrinologica* 41 (1962): 400-406.

38. Coodley, GO, et al. A trial of testosterone therapy for HIV-associated weight loss. *AIDS* (1997) 11(11):1347-1352.

39. Haupt, HA, et al. Anabolic steroids: A review of the literature. *Am J Sport Med* (1984) 12(6):469-484.

40. O'Shea, JP, et al. Biochemical and physical effects of an anabolic steroid in competitive swimmers and weightlifters. *Nutr Rep Int* (1970) 2:351-362.

41. Grinspoon, SÇ, et al. Body composition and endocrine function in women with acquired immunodeficiency syndrome wasting. *J Clin Endocrinol Metab* (1997) 82(5):1332-1337.

42. Grinspoon, SÇ, et al. Loss of lean body and muscle mass correlates with androgen levels in hypogonadal men with acquired immunodeficiency syndrome and wasting. *J Clin Endocrinol Metab* (1996) 81(11):4051-4058.

43. Klein, SA, et al. Substitution of testosterone in an HIV-1 positive patient with hypogonadism and wasting-syndrome led to a reduced rate of apoptosis. *Eur J Med Res* (1997) 2(1):30-32.

44. Wagner, GJ, et al. A comparative analysis of standard and alternative antidepressants in the treatment of human immunodeficiency virus. *Compr Psychiatry* (1996) 37(6):402-408.

45. Dickerman, RD, et al., Anabolic steroid-induced hepatotoxicity: is it overstated? *Clin J Sport Med* (1999) 9(1):34-39.

46. Poretsky, L, et al. Testicular dysfunction in human immunodeficiency virus-infected men. *Metabol* (1995) 44(7):946-953.

47. Dobs, AS, et al. Endocrine disorders in men infected with human immunodeficiency virus. *Am J Med* (1988) 84(3, pt 2):611-661.

48. Laudat, A, et al. Changes in systemic gonadal and adrenal steroids in asymptomatic human immunodeficiency virus-infected men: relationship with the CD4 T-cell counts. *Eur J Endocrinol* (1995) 133(4):418-424.

49. Dobs, AS, et al. Serum hormones in men with human immunodeficiency virus-associated wasting. *J Clin Endocrinol Metab* (1996) 81(11):4108-4112.

50. Bhasin, S. Clinical Review — Androgen treatment of hypogonadal men. *J Clin Endocrinol Metab* (1992) 74(6):1221-1225.

51. Sanford, LM. Evidence that estrogen regulation of testosterone secretion in adult rams is mediated by both indirect (gonadrotropin dependent) and direct (gonadotropin independent) means. *J Androl* (1985) 6:306-314.

52. Harman, M, et al. Reproductive hormones in aging men. Measurement of sex steroids, luteinizing hormone, and leydig cell

response to human chorionic gonadotropin. *J Clin Endocrinol Metab* (1980) 51(1):3540.

53. Burge, MR, et al. Idiopathic hypogonadotropic hypogonadism in a male runner is reversed by clomiphene citrate. *Fertil Steril* (1997) 67(4):783-785.

54. Ronnberg, L, et al. Clomiphene citrate administration to normogonadotropic subfertile men: blood hormone changes and activation of acid phosphatase in seminal fluid. *Int J Androl* (1981) 4:372-378.

55. Lunardi-Iskandar, Y, et al. Tumorigenesis and metastasis of neoplastic Kaposi's sarcoma cell line in immunodeficient mice blocked by a human pregnancy hormone. *Nature* (1995) 375(6526):64-68.

56. Bourinbaiar, AS, et al. Anti-HIV effect of beta subunit of human chorionic gonadotropin (beta hCG) in vitro. *Immunol Lett* (1995) 44(1):13-18.

57. Wolkowitz, OM, et al. Dehydroepiandrosterone (DHEA) treatment of depression. *Biol Psych* (1997) 41:311-318.

58. Gold, J, et al. Safety and efficacy of nandrolone decanoate for treatment of wasting in patients with HIV infection. *AIDS* (1996) 10(7):745-752.

59. Schwartz, AG, et al. Cancer prevention with dehydroepiandrosterone and non-androgenic structural analogs. *J Cell Biochem Suppl* (1995) 22:210-217.

60. Henderson, E, et al. Dehydroepiandrosterone (DHEA) and synthetic DHEA analogs are modest inhibitors of HIV-1 IIIB replication. *AIDS Res Hum Retroviruses* (1992) 8(5):625-631.

61. Danenberg, HD, et al. Dehydroepiandrosterone protects mice from endotoxin toxicity and reduces tumor necrosis factor production. *Antimicrob Agents Chemother* (1992) 36(10):2275-2279.

62. Yang, JY, et al. Inhibition of 3'azido-3'deoxythymidine-resistant HIV-1 infection by dehydroepiandrosterone in vitro. *Biochem Biophys Res Commun* (1994) Jun 30; 201(3):1424-1432.

63. Jacobson, MA, et al. Decreased serum dehydroepiandrosterone is associated with an increased progression of human immunodeficiency virus infection in men with CD4 cell counts of 200-499. *J Infect Dis* (1991) 164(5):864-868.

64. Nestler, JE, et al. Dehydroepiandrosterone reduces serum low density lipoprotein levels and body fat but does not alter insulin sensitivity in normal men. *J Clin Endocrinol Metab* (1988) 66(1):57-61.

65. Morales, AJ, et al. Effects of replacement dose of dehydroepiandrosterone in men and women of advancing age. *J Clin Endocrinol Metab* (1994) 78(6):1360-1367.

66. Boccuzzi, G, et al. Dehydroepiandrosterone antiestrogenic action through receptor in MCF-7 human breast cancer cell line. *Anticancer Res* (1993) 13(6A):2267-2273.

67. Simpkins, JW, et al. Variable effects of testosterone on dopamine activity in several microdissected regions in the preoptic area and medial basal hypothalamus. *Endocrinol* (1983) 112(2):665-669.

68. Wehling, M. Looking beyond the dogma of genomic steroid action: insights and facts of the 1990's. *J Mol Med* (1995) 73(9):439-447.

69. Ritchie, WP, Jr. Other causes of GI musosal injury: upper intestinal content. *Clin Invest Med* (1987) 10(3):264-269.

70. Schambelan, M, et al. Recombinant human growth hormone in patients with HIV-associated wasting: a randomized placebo-controlled trial. *Ann Intern Med* (1996) 125(11):873-882.

71. Strain, G, et al. The relationship between serum levels of insulin and sex hormone-binding globulin in men: the effect of weight loss. *J Clin Endocrinol Metab* (1994) 79(4):1173-1176.

72. Bhasin, S, et al. The effect of supraphysiological doses of testosterone on muscle size and strength in normal men. *N Engl J Med* (1996) Jul 4; 335(1):1-7.

73. Hellerstein, MK, et al. Increased de novo hepatic lipogenesis in human immunodefi-

ciency virus infection. *J Clin Endocrinol Metab* (1993) 76(3):559-565.

74. Prang, E, et al. L-glutamine promotes gain in weight and body cell mass in patients with AIDS. International Conference on AIDS Wasting (1997).

75. Hankard, RG, et al. Effect of glutamine on leucine metabolism in humans. *Am J Physiol* (1996) 271(4, pt 1):E748-E754.

76. Hickson, RC, et al. Glutamine prevents down-regulation of myosin heavy chain synthesis and muscle atrophy from glucocorticoids. *Am J Physiol* (1995) 268(4, pt 1):E730-E734.

77. Jeevanandam, M, et al. Altered lipid kinetics in adjuvant recombinant human growth hormone-treated multiple-trauma patients. *Am J Physiol* (1994) 267(4, pt 1):E560-E565.

78. Rodgers, BD, et al. Catabolic hormones and growth hormone resistance in acquired immunodeficiency syndrome and other catabolic states. *Proceedings of the Society of Experimental Biology and Medicine* (1996) Sep; 212(4):324-331.

79. Horikawa, R, et al. Growth hormone and insulin-like growth factor I stimulate Leydig cell steroidogenesis. *Eur J Pharmacol* (1989) 166(1):87-94.

80. Sherwin, BB, et al. Androgen enhances sexual motivation in females: a prospective, crossover study of sex steroid administration in the surgical menopause. *Psychosom Med* (1985) 47(4):339-351.

81. Kaplan, HS, et al. The female androgen deficiency syndrome. *J Sex Marital Ther* (1993) 19(1):3-24.

82. Friedl, KE, et al. Comparison of the effects of high dose testosterone and 19-nortestosterone to a replacement dose of testosterone on strength and body composition in normal men. *J Steroid Biochem Mol Biol* (1991) 40(4-6):607-612.

83. Rabkin, JG, et al. Testosterone replacement therapy in HIV illness. *Gen Hosp Psychiatry* 1995 Jan; 17(1):37-42.

84. *Veterinary Report: Winstrol-V Toxicology Study*, Sanofi Winthrop Inc., Animal Health Division, McPherson, KS. April 1995.

85. Skubitz, KM, et al. Oral glutamine to prevent chemotherapy induced stomatitis: a pilot study. *J Lab Clin Med* (1996) 127(2):223-228.

86. Li, J, et al. Effect of glutamine-enriched total parenteral nutrition on small intestinal gut-associated lymphoid tissue and upper respiratory tract immunity. *Surgery* (1997) 121(5):542-549.

87. Hong, RW, et al. Glutamine preserves liver glutathione after lethal hepatic injury. *Ann Surg* (1992) 215(2):114-119.

89. Wolf, RF, et al. Growth hormone and insulin reverse net whole body and skeletal muscle protein catabolism in cancer patients. *Ann Surg* (1992) 216(3):280-290.

90. Wolf, RF, et al. Growth hormone and insulin combine to improve whole-body and skeletal muscle protein kinetics. *Surgery* (1992) 112(2):284-292.

91. Roos, N, et al. 15N-labeled immunoglobulins from bovine colostrum are partially resistant to digestion in human intestine. *J Nutr* (1995) 125(5):1238-1244.

92. Bogstedt, AK, et al. Passive immunity against diarrhoea. *Acta Paediatr* (1996) 85(2):125-128.

93. Severson, K, et al. Free testosterone as a predictor for body composition changes in males with HIV or AIDS. XI International Conference on AIDS, Vancouver (1996) 11(1):332. Abstract No. Tu.B.2385.

94. Simpkins, JW, et al. Variable effects of testosterone on dopamine activity in several microdissected regions in the preoptic area and medial basal hypothalamus. *Endocrinol* (1983) 112(2):665-669.

95. Marquardt, GH, et al. Failure of non-17-alkylated steroids to produce abnormal liver function tests. *J Clin Endocrinol* (1964) 24:1334-1336.

96. Poles, MA, et al. Oxandrolone as a treatment for AIDS-related weight loss and

wasting. 4th Conference on Retroviruses and Opportunistic Infections (1997) Jan 22-26:193. Abstract No. 695.

97. Jones, JA, et al. Use of DHEA in a patient with advanced prostate cancer: a case report and review. *Urology* (1997) 50(5):784-788.

98. Bucher, G, et al. A prospective study on the safety and effect of nandrolone decanoate in HIV-positive patients. XI International Conference on AIDS, Vancouver (1996) 11(1):26. Abstract No. Mo.B.423.

99. Strawford, A, et al. Effects of nandrolone decanoate (ND) on nitrogen balance, metabolism, body composition and function in men with AIDS wasting syndrome (AWS). 2nd International Conference on Nutrition and HIV Infection, Cannes, France (1997):267.

100. Hengge, UR, et al. Oxymetholone promotes weight gain in patients with advanced human immunodeficiency virus infection. *Brit J Nutr* (1996) 75:129-138.

101. Clark, RA, et al. Clinical manifestations and predictors of survival in older women infected with HIV. *J AIDS Hum Retro* (1997) 15(5):341-345.

102. Kurz, EM, et al. Androgens regulate the dendritic length of mammalian motoneurons in adulthood. *Science* (1986) 232:395-398.

103. Welder, AA, et al. Toxic effects of anabolic-androgenic steroids in primary rat hepatic cell cultures. *J Pharmacol Toxicol Methods* (1995) 33(4):187-195.

104. Bolin, T, et al. Decreased lysophospholipase and increased phospholipase A2 activity in ileal mucosa from patients with Crohn's disease. *Digestion* (1984) 29(1):55-59.

105. Weisser, B, et al. Oxidized low-density lipoproteins in atherogenesis: possible mechanisms of action. *J Cardiovasc Pharmacol* (1992) 19 (suppl 2):S4-S7.

106. Salvato, P, et al. Conference on Nutrition and HIV Infection Cannes, France (1997) April 23-24; Abstract No. 0-003.

107. Lemon, PW, et al. Do athletes need more dietary protein and amino acids? *Int J Sports Nutri* (1995) 5;S39-S61.

108. Lemon, PW, et al. Protein requirements and muscle mass.strength changes during inensive training in novice bodybuilders. *J Appl Physiol* (1992) 73(2):767-775.

109. Chan JM, et al. Plasma insulin-like growth factor-1 and prostate cancer risk: A prospective study. *Science* (1998) 23;279:563-566.

110. Björntorp, P. The regulation of adipose tissue distribution in humans. *Int J Obes Relat Metab Disord* (1996) 20(4):291-302.

111. Yarasheski, KE, et al. Effect of growth hormone and resistance exercise on muscle growth in young men. *Am J Physiol* (1992) 262 (Endocrinol Metab 25): E261-E267.

112. Rudman D, et al. Effects of human growth hormone in men over 60 years old [see comments]. *N Engl J Med* (1990) 323(1):1-6 1990.

113. Allen, RE, et al. Regulation of skeletal muscle satellite cell proliferation and differentiation by transforming growth factor-beta, insulin-like growth factor I, and fibroblast growth factor. *J Cell Physiol* (1989) 138(2):311-315.

114. Hunt, CD, et al. Effects of dietary zinc depletion on seminal volume and zinc loss, serum testosterone concentrations, and sperm morphology in young men. *Am J Clin Nutr* (1992) Jul; 56(1): 148-157.

115. Akaza, N, et al. Effects of vitamin A deficiency on the function of the pituitary-gonadal system in male rats. *Nippon Juigaku Zasshi* (1989) Dec; 51(6):1209-1217.

116. Sanchez-Capelo, A, et al. Potassium regulates plasma testosterone and renal ornithine decarboxylase in mice. *FEBS Lett* (1993) Oct. 25; 333(1-2):32-34.

117. Berger, JR, et al. Oxandrolone in AIDS-wasting myopathy. *AIDS* (1996) Dec; 10:1657-1662.

118. Ahmed, SR, et al. Transdermal testosterone therapy in the treatment of male hypogonadism. *J Clin Endocrinol Metab* (1988) 66(3):546-551.

119. Svetec, DA, et al. The effect of parenteral testosterone replacement on prostate specific antigen in hypogonadal men with erectile dysfunction. *J Urol* (1997) 158(5):1775-1777.

120. Douglas, TH, et al. Effect of exogenous testosterone replacement on prostate-specific antigen and prostate-specific membrane antigen levels in hypogonadal men. *J Surg Oncol* (1995) 59(4):246-250.

121. Funk, KF et al. Modification of the recovery of reserpine-induced amine depletion. *Biomed Biochim Acta* (1983) 42(10):1347-1348.

122. Hannan, CJ, et al. Psychological and serum homovanillic acid changes in men administered androgenic steroids. *Psycho-neuroendocrinology* (1991) 16(4):335-343.

123. Vermes, I, et al. Action of androgenic steroids on brain neurotransmitters in rats. *Neuroendocrinology* (1979) 28(6):386-393.

124. Dieterich, D, et al. Incidence of body habitus changes in a cohort of 700 HIV-infected patients. *Infect Diseases Soc Amer* (1998) Nov 12 - 15. Abstract No. 477.

125. Torres, RA, et al. Treatment of dorsocervical fat pads (buffalo hump) and truncal obesity with Serostim (recombinant human growth hormone) in patients with AIDS maintained on HAART. XII International AIDS Conference, Geneva (1998) June 28-July 3. Abstract No. 32164.

126. Fu, YK, et al. Growth hormone augments superoxide anion secretion of human neutrophils by binding to the prolactin receptor. *J Clin Invest* (1992) 89(2):451-457.

127. Smith, JA. Neutrophils, host defense, and inflammation: a double-edged sword. *J Leukoc Biol* (1994) 56(6):672-686.

128. Weissmann, G, et al. Neutrophils: release of mediators of inflammation with special reference to rheumatoid arthritis. *Ann N Y Acad Sci* (1982) 389:11-24.

129. Fuh, G et al. Prolactin receptor antagonists that inhibit the growth of breast cancer cell lines. *J Biol Chem* (1995) 270(22):1313-1317.

130. Morales, AJ, et al. The effect of six months treatment with a 100 mg daily dose of dehydroepiandrosterone (DHEA) on circulating sex steroids, body composition and muscle strength in age-advanced men and women. *Clin Endocrinol* (Oxf) (1998) 49(4):421-432.

131. Kruskemper, HL. *Anabolic Steroids*. Academic Press (NY/London) (1968):59.

132. Kochakian, CD. Personal communication to Michael Mooney, 1995.

133. G'omez de Segura, IA, et al. Comparative effects of growth hormone in large and small bowel resection in the rat. *J Surg Res* (1996) 62(1):5-10.

134. Berni Canani, R, et al. Comparative effects of growth hormone on water and ion transport in rat jejunum, ileum, and colon. *Dig Dis Sci* (1996) 41(6):1076-1081.

135. Yarasheski, KE, et al. Effect of resistance exercise and growth hormone on bone density in older men. *Clin Endocrinol* (Oxf) (1997) 47(2):223-229.

136. Zachwieja, JJ, et al. Growth hormone administration in older adults: effects on albumin synthesis. *Am J Physiol* (1994) 266(6 Pt 1):E840-844.

137. Yarasheski, KE, et al. Effect of growth hormone and resistance exercise on muscle growth and strength in older men. *Am J Physiol* (1995) 268(2 Pt 1):E268-276.

138. Zachwieja, JJ, et al. Does growth hormone therapy in conjunction with resistance exercise increase muscle force production and muscle mass in men and women aged 60 years or older? *Phys Ther* (1999) 79(1):76-82.

139. Yarasheski, KE, et al. Growth hormone effects on metabolism, body composition,

muscle mass, and strength. *Exerc Sport Sci Rev* (1994) 22():285-312.

140. Suzuki, K, et al. Endocrine environment of benign prostatic hyperplasia: prostate size and volume are correlated with serum estrogen concentration. *Scand JUrol Nephrol* (1995) 29:65-68.

141. Gann, PH, et al. A prospective study of plasma hormone levels, nonhormonal factors, and development of benign prostatic hyperplasia. *The Prostate* (1995) 26:40-49.

142. Wagner, GJ, et al. Testosterone therapy for clinical symptoms of hypogonadism in eugonadal men with AIDS. *Int J STD & AIDS* (1998) 9:a1119.1-a1119.4.

143. Strawford, A, et al. Resistance exercise and supraphysiologic androgen therapy in eugonadal men with HIV-related weight loss. *JAMA* (1999) 281(14):1282-1290.

144. Mulligan, K, et al. Anabolic effects of recombinant human growth hormone in patients with wasting associated with human immunodeficiency virus infection. *J Clin Endocrinol Metab* (1993) 77(4):956-962.

145. Solerte, SB, et al. Hormonal and chronobiological impairment of GH-IGF1-IGFBP3 axis in HIV infected patients (CDC C3) with wasting syndrome. Effects of treatment with recombinant human GH. XI International AIDS Conference, Vancouver (1996) Abstract No. Mo. B.420.

146. Stoll, BA. Breast cancer risk in Japanese women with special reference to the growth hormone-insulin-like growth factor axis. *Jpn J Clin Oncol* (1992) Feb; 22(1):1-5.

147. Westley, BR, et al. Role of insulin-like growth factors in steroid modulated proliferation. *J Ster Biochem Mol Biol* (1994) Oct; 51(1-2):1-9.

148. Malozowski, S. et al. Prepubertal gynecomastia during growth hormone therapy. *J Pediatr* (1995) 126(4):659-661.

149. Cohn, L, et al. Carpal tunnel syndrome and gynaecomastia during growth hormone treatment of elderly men with low

circulating IGF-I concentrations. *Clin Endocrinol* (Oxf) (1993) 39(4):417-425.

150. Fuh, G, et al. Prolactin receptor antagonists that inhibit the growth of breast cancer cell lines. *J Biol Chem* (1995) 270(22):1313-1317.

Orthomolecular Nutrition

1. Lashner, BA, et al. The effect of folic acid supplementaion on the risk of cancer or dysplasia in ulcerative colitis. *Gastroenterol* (1997) 112:29-32.

2. Loriaux, SM, et al. The effect of nicotinic acid and xanthinol nicotinate on human memory in different categories of age. *Psychopharmacol* (1985) 87:390-395.

3. Stone, MH, et al. Effects of vitamin C on cortisol and the testosterone to cortisol ratio. (1995). Unpublished study of the US National Weight Lifting Team.

4. Liakakos, D, et al. Inhibitory effect of ascorbic acid on cortisol secretion following adrenal stimulation in children. *Clinical Chem Acta* (1975) 65:251-258.

5. Volek, JS, et al. Testosterone and cortisol in relationship to dietary nutrients and resistance exercise. *J Appl Physiol* (1997) 82(1):49-54.

6. Caughey, GE, et al. The effect on human tumor necrosis factor alpha and interleukin 1 beta production of diets enriched in n-3 fatty acids from vegetable oil or fish oil. *Am J Clin Nutr* (1996) 63(1):116-122.

7. Souba, WW, et al. Anabolic steroids support postoperative gut/liver amino acid metabolism. *J Parent Ent Nutr* (1988) 12(6):550-554.

8. Paavonen, T, et al. Sex hormone regulation of in vitro immune response. Estradiol enhances human B cell maturation via inhibition of suppressor T cells in pokeweed mitogen-stimulated cultures. *J Exp Med* (1981) 154(6):1935-1945.

9. Feigen, GA, et al. Sex hormones and the immune response. Host factors in the production of penicillin-specific antibodies in

the female guinea pig. *Int Arch Allergy Appl Immunol* (1978) 57(5): 385-398.

10. Munster, AM, et al. The effect of antibiotics on cell-mediated immunity. *Surgery* (1977) 81(6): 692-695.

11. Eaton, SB, et al. Paleolithic nutrition. A consideration of its nature and current implications. *N Eng J Med* (1985) 312(5): 283-289.

12. Hubbard, L, et al. *Lifeline;* Loma Linda University (1990) 5:6.

13. Hum, S. Varied protein intake alters glutathione metabolism in rats. *J Nutri* (1992) 122(10):2010-2018.

14. Lemon, PW, et al. Do athletes need more dietary protein and amino acids? *Int J Sports Nutri* (1995) 5:S39-S61.

15. Freed, DJ, et al. Anabolic steroids in athletics: crossover double-blind trial on weightlifters. *Br Med J* (1975) 2(59):471-473.

16. Zambelli, et al. Effect of two different diets on AIDS patients' nutritional status. Xl International AIDS Conference, Vancouver (1996) Abstract Th.B.4243.

17. Baum, M, et al. Inadequate dietary intake and altered nutrition status in early HIV-1 infection. *Nutrition* (1994) 10(1):16-20.

18. Abrams, B, et al. A prospective study of dietary intake and AIDS in HIV-positive homosexual men. *J AIDS* (1993) 6:949-958.

19. Baum, MK, et al. Micronutrients and HIV-1 disease progression. *AIDS* (1995) 9(9):1051-1056.

20. Tang, AM, et al. Low serum vitamin B-12 concentrations are associated with faster human immunodeficiency virus type 1 (HIV-1) disease progression. *J Nutr* (1997) 127(2):345-351.

21. Tang, AM, et al. Effects of micronutrient intake on survival in human immunodeficiency virus type 1 infection. *Am J Epidem* (1996) 143(12):1244.

22. Koch, J, et al. Zinc levels and infections in hospitalized patients with AIDS. *Nutrition* (1996) 12(7-8):515-518.

23. Mocchegiani, E, et al. Benefit of oral zinc supplementation as an adjunct to zidovu-dine (AZT) therapy against opportunistic infections in AIDS. *Int J Immunopharmacol* (1995) 17(9):719-727.

24. Baum, MK, et al. Risk of HIV-related mortality is associated with selenium deficiency. *J AIDS Hum Retro* (1997) 15:370-376.

25. Floyd, JC, et al. Stimulation of insulin secretion by amino acids. *J Clin Invest* (1966) Sep 45:1487.

26. Young, SN, et al. Folic acid and psychopathology. *Prog Neuropsychopharmacol Biol Psychiatry* (1989) 13(6):841-863.

27. Gallagher, PM, et al. Homocysteine and risk of premature coronary heart disease. Evidence for a common gene mutation. *Circulation* (1996) 94(9):2154-2158.

28. Anderson, RA, et al. Elevated intake of supplemental chromium improve glucose and insulin variables in individuals with type 2 diabetes. Diabetes (1997) 46:1786-1791.

29. Boelaert, JR, et al. Altered iron metabolism in HIV infection: mechanisms, possible consequences, and proposals for management. *Inf Agents & Dis* (1996) 5(1):36-46.

30. Omara, FO, et al. Vitamin E is protective against iron toxicity and iron-induced hepatic vitamin E depletion in mice. *J Nutrition* (1993) Oct; 123(10):1649-1655.

31. Dworkin, BM, et al. Abnormalities of blood selenium and glutathione peroxidase activity in patients with acquired immunodeficiency syndrome and AIDS-related complex. *Biol Trace Elem Res* (1988) 15():167-177.

32. Meydani, SN, et al. Vitamin E supplementation and in vivo immune response in healthy elderly subjects. A randomized controlled trial. *J Am Med Assoc* (1997) 277:1380-1386.

33. Devaraj, S, et al. The effects of alpha tocopherol supplementation on monocyte function: decreased lipid oxidation, interleukin 1 beta secretion, and monocyte adhesion to endothelium. *J Clin Invest* (1996) 98(3):756-763.

34. Busse, E, et al. Influence of alpha-lipoic acid on intracellular glutathione in vitro

and in vivo. *Arzneimittel-Forshung* (1992) 42;829-831.

35. Herzenberg L, et al. Glutathione deficiency is associated with impaired survival in HIV disease. *Proceedings of the National Academy of Sciences USA* (1997) 94(5):1967-1972.

36. Packer, L, et al. Neuroprotection by the metabolic antioxidant a-lipoic acid. *Free Rad Biol & Med* (1997) 22(1/2):359-378.

37. Semba, RD, et al. Increased mortality associated with vitamin A deficiency during human immunodeficiency virus type 1 infection. *Arch Intern Med* (1993) 153(18):2149-2154.

38. Tang, AM, et al. Association between serum vitamin A and E levels and HIV-1 disease progression. *AIDS* (1997) 11(5):613-620.

39. Greenberg, BL, et al. Vitamin A deficiency and maternal-infant transmissions of HIV in two metropolitan areas in the United States. *AIDS* (1997) 11(3):325-332.

40. Beach, RS, et al. Plasma vitamin B12 level as a potential cofactor in studies of human immunodeficiency virus type 1-related cognitive changes. *Arch Neurol* (1992) 49(5):501-506.

41. Sprince, H, et al. Protection against acetaldehyde toxicity in the rat by L-cysteine, thiamin and L-2-methylthiazolidine-4-carboxylic acid. *Agents Actions* (1974) 4(2):125-130.

42. Estrela, JM, et al. The effect of cysteine and N-acetyl cysteine on rat liver glutathione (GSH). *Biochem Pharmacol* (1983)32(22):3483-3485.

43. Bogden, JD, et al. Daily micronutrient supplements enhance delayed-hypersensitivity skin test responses in older people. *Am J Clin Nutr* (1994) 60(3):437-447.

44. Chandra, RK, et al. Effect of vitamin and trace-element supplementation on immune responses and infection in elderly subjects. *Lancet* (1992) 340 (8828):1124-1127.

44. Hellerstein, MK, et al. Effects of dietary n-3 fatty acid supplementation in men with weight loss associated with the acquired immune deficiency syndrome: relation to indices of cytokine production. *J AIDS Hum Retro* (1996)11(3):258-270.

45. De Simone, C, et al. High dose L-carnitine improves immunologic and metabolic parameters in AIDS patients. *Immunopharmacol Immunotoxicol* (1993) 15(1):1-12.

46. Rai, G, et al. Double-blind, placebo controlled study of acetyl-l-carnitine in patients with Alzheimer's dementia. *Curr Med Res Opin* (1990) 11(10):638-647.

47. Oda, T, et al. Effect of lactobacillus acidophilus on iron bioavailability in rats. *J Nutr Sci Vitaminol* (Tokyo) (1994) 40(6):613-616.

48. Bishinell, MF. *Lancet* (1952)11:53.

49. De Flora, S, et al. Attenuation of influenza-like symptomology and improvement of cell-mediated immunity with long-term N-acetylcysteine treatment. *Euro Respir Journal* (1997) 10:1535-1541.

50. Biolo, G, et al. An abundant supply of amino acids enhances the metabolic effect of exercise on muscle protein. *Am J Phys* (1997) 36:E122-E129.

51. Okamura, K, et al. Effect of amino acid and glucose administration during post exercise recovery on protein kinetics in dogs. *Am J Physiol* (1997) 272(6, pt 1): E1023-E1030.

52. Hong, RW, et al. Glutamine preserves liver glutathione after lethal hepatic injury. *Ann Surg* (1992) 215(2):114-119.

53. Hickson, RC, et al. Glutamine prevents downregulation of myosin heavy chain synthesis and muscle atrophy from glucocorticoids. *Am J Physiol* (1995) 268 (4, pt 1): E730-E734.

54. Hankard, RG, et al. Effect of glutamine on leucine metabolism in humans. *Am J Physiol* (1996) 271(4, pt 1):E748-E754.

55. Li, J, et al. Effect of glutamine-enriched total parenteral nutrition on small intestinal gut-associated lymphoid tissue and upper

respiratory tract immunity. *Surgery* (1997) 121(5):542-549.

56. Ardawi, MS, et al. Glutamine metabolism in lymphocytes and its importance in the immune response. *Essays in Biochemistry* (1985).

57. Anon. Muscle provides glutamine to the immune system. *Nutr Rev.* (1990) 48:390-392.

58. Skubitz, KM, et al. Oral glutamine to prevent chemotherapy-induced stomatitis: a pilot study. *J Lab Clin Med* (1996) 127(2):223-228.

59. Prang, E, et al. L-glutamine promotes gain in weight and body cell mass in patients with AIDS. International Conference on AIDS Wasting (1997).

60. Sprince H, et al. Protective action of ascorbic acid and sulfur compounds against acetaldehyde toxicity: implications in alcoholism and smoking. *Agents Actions* (1975) 5(2):164-273.

61. Boirie, Y, et al. Slow and fast dietary proteins differently modulate postprandial protein accretion. *Proceedings of the National Academy of Sciences USA* (1997) 94:14930-14935.

62. Ferenci P, et al. Randomized controlled trial of silymarin treatment in patients with cirrhosis of the liver. *J Hepatol* (1989) 9:105-113.

63. Hikino H, et al. *Planta Medica* (1984) 50: 248-250.

64. Wagner, H. Plant constituents with anti-hepatotoxic activity. In: Beal, J., & Reinhard, E., eds. Natural Products as Medicinal Agents (Stuttgart, Germany) Hippokrates-Verlag (1981) pp. 545-558.

65. Bounous, G, et al. Whey protein as a food supplement in HIV-seropositive individuals. *Clin & Invest Med* (1993) Jun; 16(3): 204-209.

66. Bounous, G, et al. Immunoenhancing property of dietary whey protein in mice: role of glutathione. *Clin & Invest Med* (1989) 12:154-161.

67. Bounous, G, et al. The biological activity of undenatured dietary whey proteins: the role of glutathione. *Clin & Invest Med* (1991) 14(4):296-309.

68. Truswell, AS. Food carbohydrates and plasma lipids — an update. *Am J Clin Nutr* (1994) 59(suppl 3):S710-S718.

69. Miller, JC, et al. Replacing starch with sucrose in a high glycaemic index breakfast cereal lowers glycaemic and insulin responses. *Eur J Clin Nutr* (1994) 48(10):749-752.

70. den Heijer, M, et al. Vitamin supplementation reduces blood homocysteine levels: a controlled trial in patients with venous thrombosis and healthy volunteers. *Arterioscler Thromb Vasc Biol* (1998) 18(3):356-361.

71. Mantero-Atienza, E, et al. Vitamin B6 and immune function in HIV infection. VI International Conference on AIDS (1990) 6(2):432 Abstract No. 3123.

72. Tang, AM, et al. The effect of micronutrient intake on survival in HIV-1 infection. XI International Conference on AIDS, Vancouver (1994) 10(2):220. Abstract No. PB0894.

73. Shor-Posner, G, et al. Anxiety and depression in early HIV-1 infection and its association with vitamin B6 status. VIII International Conference on AIDS (1992) 8(2):B209. Abstract No. POB 3711.

74. Ubbink, JB, et al. The effect of a subnormal vitamin B-6 status on homocysteine metabolism. *J Clin Invest* (1996) 98(1):177-184.

75. Famularo, G, et al. Acetyl-carnitine deficiency in AIDS patients with neurotoxicity on treatment with antiretroviral nucleoside analogues. *AIDS* (1997) 11(2):185-190.

76. Lowitt, S, et al. Acetyl-L-carnitine corrects the altered peripheral nerve function of experimental diabetes. *Metabolism* (1995) 44(5):677-680.

77. Faure, P, et al. Vitamin E improves the free radical defense system potential and insulin sensitivity of rats fed high fructose diets. *J Nutr* (1997) 127(1):103-107.

78. Basualdo, CG, et al. Vitamin A (retinol) status of first nation adults with non-insulin-

dependent diabetes mellitus. *J Am Coll Nutr* (1997) 16(1):39-45.

79. Sanchez, M. et al. Oral calcium supplementation reduces intraplatelet free calcium concentration and insulin resistance in essential hypertensive patients. *Hypertension* (1997) 29(1 Pt 2):531-536.

80. Moretti, S, et al. Effect of L-carnitine on human immunodeficiency virus-1 infection-associated apoptosis: a pilot study. *Blood* (1998) 91(10):3817-3824.

81. Fernandez-Real, JM, et al. Serum ferritin as a component of the insulin resistance syndrome. *Diabetes Care* (1998) 21(1):62-68.

82. Nestler, JE, et al. Dehydroepiandrosterone reduces serum low density lipoprotein levels and body fat but does not alter insulin sensitivity in normal men. *J Clin Endocrinol Metab* (1988) 66(1):57-61.

83. Morales, AJ, et al. Effects of replacement dose of dehydroepiandrosterone in men and women of advancing age. *J Clin Endocrinol Metab* (1994) 78(6):1360-1367.

84. Wolkowitz, OM, et al. Dehydroepiandrosterone (DHEA) treatment of depression. *Biol Psych* (1997) 41:311-318.

85. Schwartz, AG, et al. Cancer prevention with dehydroepiandrosterone and non-androgenic structural analogs. *J Cell Biochem Suppl* (1995) 22:210-217.

86. Henderson, E, et al. Dehydroepiandrosterone (DHEA) and synthetic DHEA analogs are modest inhibitors of HIV-1 IIIB replication. *AIDS Res Hum Retroviruses* (1992) 8(5):625-631.

87. Danenberg, HD, et al. Dehydroepiandrosterone protects mice from endotoxin toxicity and reduces tumor necrosis factor production. *Antimicrob Agents Chemother* (1992) 36(10):2275-2279.

88. Yang, JY, et al. Inhibition of 3'azido-3'deoxythymidine-resistant HIV-1 infection by dehydroepiandrosterone in vitro. *Biochem Biophys Res Commun* (1994) Jun 30; 201(3):1424-1432.

89. Jacobson, MA, et al. Decreased serum dehydroepiandrosterone is associated with an increased progression of human immunodeficiency virus infection in men with CD4 cell counts of 200-499. *J Infect Dis* (1991) 164(5):864-868.

90. Jones, JA, et al. Use of DHEA in a patient with advanced prostate cancer: a case report and review. *Urology* (1997) 50(5):784-788.

91. Boccuzzi, G. et al. Dehydroepiandrosterone antiestrogenic action through receptor in MCF-7 human breast cancer cell line. *Anticancer Res* (1993) 13(6A):2267-2273.

92. Laudat, A, et al. Changes in systemic gonadal and adrenal steroids in asymptomatic human immunodeficiency virus-infected men: relationship with the CD4 T cell counts. *Eur J Endocrinol* (1995) 133(4):418-424.

93. Simpkins, JW, et al. Variable effects of testosterone on dopamine activity in several microdissected regions in the preoptic area and medial basal hypothalamus. *Endocrinol* (1983) 112(2):665-669.

94. Wehling, M. Looking beyond the dogma of genomic steroid action: insights and facts of the 1990's. *J Mol Med* (1995) 73(9):439-447.

95. Wolf, RF, et al. Growth hormone and insulin reverse net whole body and skeletal muscle protein catabolism in cancer patients. *Ann Surg* (1992) 216(3):280-290.

96. Ritchie, WP, Jr. Other causes of GI musosal injury: upper intestinal content. *Clin Invest Med* (1987) 10(3):264-269.

97. Bolin, T, et al. Decreased lysophospholipase and increased phospholipase A2 activity in ileal mucosa from patients with Crohn's disease. *Digestion* (1984) 29(1):55-59.

98. Weisser, B, et al. Oxidized low-density lipoproteins in atherogenesis: possible mechanisms of action. *J Cardiovasc Pharmacol* (1992) 19 (suppl 2):S4-S7.

99. Kremer, JM, et al. Dietary fish oil and olive oil supplementation in patients with rheumatoid arthritis. Clinical and immunologic effects. *Athritis Rheum* (1990) 33(6):810-820.

100. Franken, DG, et al. Treatment of mild hyperhomocysteinemia in vascular disease patients. *Arterioscler Thromb* (1994) 14(3):465-470.

101. Dandona, P, et al. Insulin resistance and iron overload. *Ann Clin Biochem* (1983) 20 Pt 2():77-79.

102. Akaza, N, et al. Effects of vitamin A deficiency on the function of the pituitary-gonadal system in male rats. *Nippon Juigaku Zasshi* (1989) Dec;51(6):1209-1217.

103. Evain-Brion, D, et al. Vitamin A deficiency and nocturnal growth hormone secretion in short children. *The Lancet* (1994) 343:87-88.

104. Hunt, CD, et al. Effects of dietary zinc depletion on seminal volume and zinc loss, serum testosterone concentrations, and sperm morphology in young men. *Am J Clin Nutr* (1992) Jul;56(1):148-157.

105. Dorup, A, et al. Role of insulin-like growth factor-1 and growth hormone in growth inhibition induced by magnesium and zinc deficiencies. *Br J Nutr* (1991) Nov;66(3):505-521.

106. Hadjivassiliou, M, et al. Does cryptic gluten sensitivity play a part in neurological illness? *Lancet* (1996) 347(8998):369-371.

107. Allard, JP, et al. Effects of vitamin E and C supplementation on oxidative stress and viral load in HIV-infected subjects. AIDS (1998) 12(13):1653-1659.

Pediatric AIDS

1. Buyukgebiz, A, et al. Treatment of constitutional delay of growth and puberty with oxandrolone compared with growth hormone. *Arch Dis Child* (1990) 65(4):448-449.

2. Howard, CP, et al. Children with growth hormone deficiency: intermittent treatment with somatropin and oxandrolone. *Am J Dis Child* (1981) 135(4):326-328.

3. Rosenfeld, RG, et al. Growth hormone therapy of Turner's syndrome: beneficial effect on adult height. *J Pediatr* (1998) 132(2):319-324.

4. Nilsson, KO, et al. Improved final height in girls with Turner's syndrome treated with growth hormone and oxandrolone. *J Clin Endocrinol Metab* (1996) 81(2):635-640.

5. Zambelli, et al. Effect of two different diets on AIDS patients' nutritional status. Xl International AIDS Conference Vancouver (1996) Abstract Th.B.4243.

6. Boirie, Y, et al. Slow and fast dietary proteins differently modulate postprandial protein accretion. *Proceedings of the National Academy of Science USA* (1997) 94: 14930-14935.

7. Bounous, G, et al. Immunoenhancing property of dietary whey protein in mice: role of glutathione. *Clin & Invest Med* (1989) 12:154-161.

8. Bounous, G, et al. The biological activity of undenatured dietary whey proteins: the role of glutathione. *Clin & Invest Med* (1991) 14(4):296-309.

9. Bogstedt, AK, et al. Passive immunity against diarrhoea. *Acta Paediatr* (1996) 85(2):125-128.

Exercise

1. Olson, PE, et al. CD4 correlates of weight-training in HIV-seropositive outpatients. 2nd Nat. Conf on Human Retroviruses and Related Infections Washington, D.C. (1995) Jan. 29-Feb 2. Abstract 544.

2. Spence, DW, et al. Progressive resistance exercise: effect on muscle function and anthropometry of a select AIDS population. *Arch Phys Med Rehabil* (1990) 71(9):644-648.

3. Rigsby, LW, et al. Effects of exercise training on men seropositive for the human immunodeficiency virus-1. *Med Sci Sports Exerc* (1992) 24(1):6-12.

PoWeR

Program for Wellness Restoration, is a grass-roots, information-based treatment and research advocacy organization. Our purpose is to disseminate empowering information to patients and healthcare professionals about a comprehensive, state-of-the-art approach to build lean body mass for optimal health and well-being. Our approach includes the medical use of anabolic steroids, and other hormonal therapies, combined with proper nutrition, dietary supplements, and resistance weight-training. PoWeR is operated primarily by volunteers and relies solely on private, tax-deductible contributions and its own fundraising efforts. PoWeR is a 501(c) 3 nonprofit corporation. PoWeR seminars are endorsed by more than 148 physicians and 100 HIV/AIDS agencies.

Your PoWeR Resources

We are here to help you learn how to stop losing lean body mass (wasting) and regain it and your health. Our resources for HIV(+) people include our telephone question and answer hotline 1(310) 360-0654, this book, our newsletter, and our national lecture series. Ask your local AIDS organization to bring us to your city to lecture.

Ordering This Book

To order copies of this book, call the Houston Buyer's Club, 1 (800) 350-2392. You can also obtain it through major book dealers like Barnes and Noble and Amazon.com.

The Medical Anabolic Newsletter — Medibolics

For a four issue subscription, send $20.00 to: Medibolics, P.O. Box # 333, 836 N. La Cienega Boulevard. West Hollywood, CA 90069. (See the Medibolics section on page 140 for information on the contents of back issues.)

Web Sites

See selected articles from Medibolics on the internet at http://www.medibolics.com. Find the PoWeR web page by going to the Medibolics web site and using the link to PoWeR.

Seminars

Call Michael or Nelson directly to discuss bringing one of them to speak in your city. Seminar events can be tailored for your organization.

PoWeR Contacts

Jim Brockman — PoWeR question and answer line: 1 (310) 360-0654

Michael Mooney, Los Angeles, 1 (310) 360-0654, FAX: 1 (310) 659-1597, e-mail: mmooney@icnt.net

Nelson Vergel, Houston, 1 (713) 520-6630, FAX: 1 (713) 526-5883, e-mail: powertx@aol.com

---

DISCLAIMER:

The information contained in this publication is for educational purposes only, and is in no way a substitute for the advice of a qualified medical doctor or a recommendation to do other than your doctor determines is best for you. You should present this information to your doctor for their analysis because appropriate medical therapy and the use of pharmaceutical compounds like anabolic steroids should be tailored by a knowledgeable doctor for the individual as no two individuals are alike. We do not recommend self-medicating with any pharmaceutical compound as you should consult with a qualified medical doctor who can determine your individual situation. Any use of the information presented in this publication for personal medical therapy is done strictly at your own risk and no responsibility is implied or intended on the part of the authors or publisher.

Personal Testimonials

The first letter is from a man who has experienced the benefits of very progressive use of anabolic steroids. Because everyone is so different, all doctors should be willing to work creatively with a patient to find what gives them optimal quality-of-life. For some people, different dosages will work better. While many men will respond to 100 to 200 mg per week of testosterone, we have seen others who are highly progressed in AIDS who do not feel normal energy levels until they were given 300 mg of testosterone along with 300 mg of nandrolone per week. Quite a difference! With a complex critical illness like HIV/AIDS there is no one-size-fits-all formula.

Dear Michael:

Back in June I asked you for a reference in New York for a doctor who would prescribe steroids to HIV patients. You sent me to Dr. Doug Dieterich. You also asked that I let you know how I liked him. I must thank you heartfully for the recommendation. Doug sat with me and listened to my story. Mine is not nearly as bad as many. I only lost one lover and one close friend. I myself only had Kaposi's sarcoma, which was "cured" with interferon three years ago. Doug said it sounded like I was depressed. I never thought of it that way. I just thought dragging my butt every day was part of the dark cloud AIDS brought with it.

Doug put me on 200 mg of testosterone and 2000 mcg of B12 immediately. I had an energy jump, not to mention the sex drive jump. For the next six weeks I was on 100 mg of testosterone per week since my testosterone levels seemed to be normal. Still my weight dropped two pounds at this dosage. I had been seeing the nutritionist attached to the clinic. Now I wanted to see the doctor again. I asked for a cycle of Deca and Doug gave me 200 mg of Deca plus 200 mg of testosterone immediately. I have not felt this together for 15 years. The drugs have taken away the looming dark cloud and have given me a greater sense of control over my body and consequently helped me to focus my life. Work is better and I have energy to get through the day and still get to the gym. I am more patient with my staff and feel a heightened sense of self esteem.

I am very pleased with what has been done at the clinic. I am not certain whether it is the drugs or the plain psychological effect of knowing that I am doing something to help my body beyond just keeping AIDS somewhat capped with protease inhibitors. Thanks for the recommendation!

L. Marks

Dear Nelson,

If you have not taken time to look around and see the impact your work has had on so many, many lives that would have been lost otherwise...please stop and notice. Your work should be getting the same press as the protease inhibitors. I believe it makes that much difference in the quality-of-life of an HIV-infected person. Thanks for showing me the way to manifest dreams. I love you, Nelson.

Arlette Pharo, DO

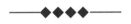

Dear PoWeR,

I have AIDS and had taken on the appearance of a holocaust victim. My lifetime normal weight of 145 lbs. had reached a low of 125 lbs. Six weeks later, following Nelson Vergel's recommended PoWeR program I weigh more now than I have ever weighed. At 150 lbs. plus, I look and feel great. One fantastic side effect has been the return of a more normal sex life.

C. Kirby

Dear PoWeR,

Over a period of approximately 10 months I was facing an ever-increasing list of symptoms including nausea and vomiting, weakness, fatigue, weight loss, and the associated depression. I was just plain sick and felt lousy, but nobody seemed to listen to me. Finally my doctor, Dr. Shannon Schrader referred me to Nelson Vergel. I spoke with Nelson and he assured me I was a good candidate for his PoWeR program for wellness restoration. He took the time to schedule an appointment in his office in Houston. Nelson was very sympathetic and really understood my frustration and failing health. At last, someone who understood! After only two weeks of following his simple program I gained 10 lbs., and had more energy than I'd had in months. I remember telling Nelson, *"my only regret is that I didn't start sooner!"* Five weeks have gone by since my initial contact with Nelson, and I have gained 19 lbs. of lean body mass, my energy level has sky-rocketed, and I have not even started working out yet. I have not felt this good in many months! As an LVN, I learned much about proper nutrition and exercise, as well as the use of steroids in some HIV wasting cases. Never had it been explained as thoroughly and simply and applied with such effectiveness, until I had the great fortune to meet Nelson Vergel and begin my own program for wellness restoration. Bravo Nelson! Thank you for giving me hope and showing me that it is possible to feel good again!

Randy C.

Dear Michael Mooney,

Thanks so much for your suggestions at the last Built To Survive lecture you gave in West Hollywood. I was the one who came up to you with all the joint and tendon problems in knees and elbows from working out. Since your talk I have added acupuncture, Knox Nutri-Joint gelatin (three scoops per day), loose glutamine (two spoonfuls per day), loose glucosamine sulfate (three or four spoons per day) and alpha lipoic acid (800 mg per day) to the regimen. I have to say that there has been phenomenal improvement in the tendonitis, numbness and ulnar nerve dysfunction in my forearms. I know the alpha lipoic acid works because when I ran out of the pills the pain returned, and it subsided when I started taking them again. I have started working out again for upper body, only two days per week, but the point is that I can work out at all. My knees are still very problematic, but I am confident that this regimen can only increase the chances of their healing more speedily.

With sincere appreciation,
P. Arenson

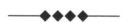

Dear Nelson,

I am an HIV-positive ..... hummmm use to think that being positive was a GOOD THING. Well, actually I still do. I have never been so alive since I discovered that I was HIV-positive a couple of years ago — decided to either get crazy and die, or GET REAL and do something fantastic to my body. I was lucky in that the new protease medication was just starting to hit the market. I had a viral load at 14000 and T4 cell count of 500. Weight was about 170 lbs., size 33 waist, however, even now without starting on the big O protease yet. I have an undetectable viral load, and T4 count of 800. 172 lbs., size 31 waist (leaner). I am taking Anadrol and working out four days each week. Was taking testosterone cypionate - a 200 mg injection once per week. My doctor suggested that I try Anadrol to see how it worked with me. I am meeting my doctor today to discuss stacking testosterone cypionate with the Anadrol as I understand that they work better together.

It is a crazy, scary world when you discover that you are HIV-positive. All doctors have different ideas on treatment. Other HIV(+) people have different suggestions for treatment, etc. It is such a wonderful thing to find someone like you folks...(Nelson Vergel)... that shed light on how we can survive - through such dedication to research done through long, hard hours. THANK YOU, THANK YOU, THANK YOU, THANK YOU.

Your hard work and the lives you save through sharing your knowledge is appreciated by us, and our friends and family that love us and want us around. You are loved.

Thanks (such a simple word for so much),

Jerry

Dear Michael,

I have taken the PoWeR suggestions for eating and steroids quite seriously for the last six months and actually have had my protease pot belly shrink down so that it's barely sticking out and my triglycerides decrease to the high end of normal. I am currently taking testosterone and Winstrol, and avoiding all sugar and starch, and will continue too, as long as it keeps working. Thank you for giving me your time and your knowledge.

Mark T.

——◆◆◆——

Guys,

I been on a Deca/testosterone regime for about 6 months, and I am very happy with it. I feel like I look like a healthy human again. I have put on about ten pounds of muscle and my face has filled out. My cheeks are still a little drawn, but with the rest of my face filling, you hardly notice it. And my butt has even returned. But most important, the crix belly has definitely gone down. People have told me I look like I have lost 10 pounds (I've gained it). I know, because my waist size has gone down. Lifting weight with some aerobics is a big part of it, along with the Deca/testosterone I have put on a total of 40 pounds.

Mark

——◆◆◆——

Nelson,

Tim here from Dallas. I spoke with you a couple of months ago. Was experiencing dramatic weight loss, dropped to 155 from 175. Started a modified PoWeR cycle. We are now at 200 mg testosterone and 100 mg nandrolone every other week. Glad I am almost done since they have stopped manufacturing the generic and the Deca is on back order. The results have been phenomenal, I am now up to 188 lbs. and have gotten noticeably bigger.

Thanks for all the help.

Tim

——◆◆◆——

BIG THANKS to Michael and Nelson for making me aware of Deca via the PoWeR web site. Last year, when I found out about PoWeR, my doctor (who is fairly progressive) had no knowledge of anabolics and I had to educate him. I told all of my friends about PoWeR. You guys have helped many people.

Cheers!
Jari D.

In the summer of 1992 I was diagnosed with HIV while pursuing a career as an actor in West Hollywood, California. My dreams seemed to vanish before me as I packed my bags and moved back to my family in Pennsylvania to await death.

Three years later I developed anemia, KS, and lymphoma as my viral load skyrocketed to 750,000 and my T cells fell to 70. Hospitalized for a month I underwent transfusions, chemotherapy and dual antiretroviral therapy. I was told I had 6 months to live. Fortunately, access to the new protease inhibitors brought my viral load down to 1,700 while my T cells rose to 250. Friends from Los Angeles told me of anabolic therapy but my doctor dismissed it as novel and unnecessary.

Determined to survive I gained access to the internet and surfed to find Medibolics. I hungrily devoured the information and decided to email Michael Mooney. Much to my surprise he emailed me back and a phone conversation soon followed. I found Michael to be the most educated and compassionate man that I have ever spoken to concerning HIV and survival. Once again empowered with an arsenal of information I was able to convince my doctor to give me a testosterone test, which showed that I was low at only 200. She put me on the ALZA patch and we both watched as my zest for life and strength increased.

Soon after this we both had the pleasure of attending a lecture in Harrisburg by Nelson Vergel, who shared his personal story and insight. We experimented with Oxandrin, and I gained more weight. Then I saw Dr. Douglas Dieterich of New York, who worked with me using Deca and testosterone with incredible success. Thanks to anabolic therapy I have my life back right where I want it. I am in the best shape of my life, I have become a personal trainer, teach aerobics 6 days per week, and my quality of life is the best ever. This empowerment to survive and the Built To Survive handbook have given me the guidelines to a healthy way of life where a person with HIV does not have to look and feel sick. Although I will always have a battle with HIV, I feel that I can meet any challenges that I have to face, and I have much to share to empower others like myself who are facing adversity.

Thank you,

Jim
Harrisburg, PA

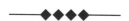

Nelson and Michael,
You are practicing what the scientists only theorize ... they can learn a lot from your hard work and from the good work of PoWeR.

Thank you,

Ed

Index